INTERVENTIONAL CARDIOLOGY CLINICS

www.interventional.theclinics.com

Editor-in-Chief

MATTHEW J. PRICE

Coronary and Endovascular Stents

July 2016 • Volume 5 • Number 3

Editor

SAHIL A. PARIKH

ELSEVIER

1600 John F. Kennedy Boulevard • Suite 1800 • Philadelphia, Pennsylvania, 19103-2899

http://www.theclinics.com

INTERVENTIONAL CARDIOLOGY CLINICS Volume 5, Number 3
July 2016 ISSN 2211-7458, ISBN-13: 978-0-323-44847-5

Editor: Lauren Boyle
Developmental Editor: Susan Showalter

Interventional Cardiology Clinics (ISSN 2211-7458) is published quarterly by Elsevier Inc., 360 Park Avenue South, New York, NY 10010-1710. Months of issue are January, April, July, and October. Subscription prices are USD 195 per year for US individuals, USD 436 for US institutions, USD 100 per year for US students, USD 195 per year for Canadian individuals, USD 520 for Canadian institutions, USD 150 per year for Canadian students, USD 295 per year for international individuals, USD 520 for international institutions, and USD 150 per year for international students. To receive student/resident rate, orders must be accompanied by name of affiliated institution, date of term, and the *signature* of program/residency coordinator on institution letterhead. Orders will be billed at individual rate until proof of status is received. Foreign air speed delivery is included in all *Clinics* subscription prices. All prices are subject to change without notice. **POSTMASTER:** Send address changes to *Interventional Cardiology Clinics*, Elsevier Health Sciences Division, Subscription Customer Service, 3251 Riverport Lane, Maryland Heights, MO 63043. **Customer Service: Telephone: 1-800-654-2452** (U.S. and Canada); **1-314-447-8871** (outside U.S. and Canada). **Fax: 1-314-447-8029. E-mail: journalscustomerservice-usa@elsevier.com (for print support); journalsonlinesupport-usa@elsevier.com (for online support).**

Reprints. For copies of 100 or more of articles in this publication, please contact the Commercial Reprints Department, Elsevier Inc., 360 Park Avenue South, New York, NY 10010-1710. Tel.: 212-633-3874; Fax: 212-633-3820; E-mail: reprints@elsevier.com.

CONTRIBUTORS

EDITOR-IN-CHIEF

MATTHEW J. PRICE, MD
Assistant Professor, Scripps Translational
Science Institute; Director of the Cardiac
Catheterization Laboratory, Scripps Green
Hospital, La Jolla, California

EDITOR

SAHIL A. PARIKH, MD, FACC, FSCAI
Director, Center for Research and Innovation,
University Hospitals Harrington Heart and
Vascular Institute; Director, Interventional
Cardiology Fellowship Program, University
Hospitals Harrington Heart and Vascular
Institute; Division of Cardiovascular Medicine,
Department of Medicine, University Hospitals
Case Medical Center, Assistant Professor of
Medicine, Case Western Reserve University
School of Medicine, Cleveland, Ohio

AUTHORS

EHRIN J. ARMSTRONG, MD, MSc
Division of Cardiology, VA Eastern Colorado
Healthcare System, University of Colorado,
Denver, Colorado

DAVIDE CAPODANNO, MD, PhD
Cardio-Thoracic-Vascular Department,
Ferrarotto Hospital, University of Catania,
Catania, Italy

ELAZER REUVEN EDELMAN, MD, PhD
Institute for Medical Engineering and Science,
Massachusetts Institute of Technology,
Cambridge, Massachusetts; Division of
Cardiovascular Medicine, Department of
Medicine, Brigham and Women's Hospital,
Harvard Medical School, Boston,
Massachusetts

JULIUS B. ELMORE, MD
Fellow, Department of Cardiology, Harrington
Heart and Vascular Institute, University
Hospitals Case Medical Center, Case Western
Reserve University School of Medicine,
Cleveland, Ohio

ALOKE VIRMANI FINN, MD
CVPath Institute Inc, Gaithersburg, Maryland;
Division of Cardiology, Department of
Medicine, University of Maryland School of
Medicine, Baltimore, Maryland

ANWER HABIB, MD
Division of Cardiology, Department of Internal
Medicine, Emory University School of
Medicine, Atlanta, Georgia

VIKRAM S. KASHYAP, MD
Chief, Department of Vascular Surgery and
Endovascular Therapy, University Hospitals
Case Medical Center, Cleveland, Ohio

JOHN H. KEATING, DVM
CBSET, Pathology, Lexington, Massachusetts

KUMARAN KOLANDAIVELU, MD, PhD
Institute for Medical Engineering and Science,
Massachusetts Institute of Technology,
Cambridge, Massachusetts; Cardiovascular
Division, Brigham and Women's Hospital,
Harvard Medical School, Boston,
Massachusetts

MARY BETH KOSSUTH, PhD
Abbott Vascular, Santa Clara, California

JUN LI, MD
Department of Medicine, Case Western
Reserve University School of Medicine,
Cleveland, Ohio; Division of Cardiovascular
Medicine, Harrington Heart and Vascular
Institute, University Hospitals Case Medical
Center, Cleveland, Ohio

EMILE MEHANNA, MD
Fellow, Department of Cardiology, Harrington
Heart and Vascular Institute, University
Hospitals Case Medical Center, Case Western
Reserve University School of Medicine,
Cleveland, Ohio

KENTA NAKAMURA, MD
CBSET, Applied Sciences, Lexington,
Massachusetts; Institute for Medical
Engineering and Science, Massachusetts
Institute of Technology, Cambridge,
Massachusetts; Division of Cardiology,
Department of Medicine, Massachusetts
General Hospital, Harvard Medical School,
Boston, Massachusetts

SAHIL A. PARIKH, MD, FACC, FSCAI
Director, Center for Research and Innovation,
University Hospitals Harrington Heart and
Vascular Institute; Director, Interventional
Cardiology Fellowship Program, University
Hospitals Harrington Heart and Vascular
Institute; Division of Cardiovascular Medicine,
Department of Medicine, University Hospitals
Case Medical Center, Assistant Professor of
Medicine, Case Western Reserve University
School of Medicine, Cleveland, Ohio

RAMON A. PARTIDA, MD
Clinical and Research Fellow, Division of
Cardiology, Department of Medicine,
Massachusetts General Hospital, Boston,
Massachusetts; Post-doctoral Research
Fellow, Institute for Medical Engineering and
Science, Massachusetts Institute of
Technology, Cambridge, Massachusetts;
Harvard Medical School, Boston,
Massachusetts

SANDEEP M. PATEL, MD
Department of Medicine, Case Western
Reserve University School of Medicine,
Cleveland, Ohio; Division of Cardiovascular
Medicine, Harrington Heart and Vascular

Institute, University Hospitals Case Medical
Center, Cleveland, Ohio

LAURA E.L. PERKINS, DVM, PhD, DACVP
Abbott Vascular, Santa Clara, California

ALEXIS POWELL, MD
Department of Vascular Surgery and
Endovascular Therapy, University Hospitals
Case Medical Center, Cleveland, Ohio

RICHARD J. RAPOZA, PhD
Abbott Vascular, Santa Clara, California

FARHAD RIKHTEGAR, PhD
Institute for Medical Engineering and Science,
Massachusetts Institute of Technology,
Cambridge, Massachusetts

RICHARD A. SCHATZ, MD
Division of Cardiology, Scripps Clinic, La Jolla,
California

CHRISTINA TAN, MD
Division of Cardiology, Scripps Clinic, La Jolla,
California

ABRAHAM RAMI TZAFRIRI, PhD
Department of Applied Sciences, CBSET,
Lexington, Massachusetts; IMES, MIT,
Cambridge, Massachusetts

STEPHEN W. WALDO, MD
Division of Cardiology, VA Eastern Colorado
Healthcare System, University of Colorado,
Denver, Colorado

DOMINIK M. WIKTOR, MD
Division of Cardiology, VA Eastern Colorado
Healthcare System, University of Colorado,
Denver, Colorado

ROBERT W. YEH, MD, MSc, MBA
Director, Department of Medicine, Smith
Center for Outcomes Research in Cardiology,
CardioVascular Institute, Beth Israel Medical
Center; Medical Director of Trial Design,
Harvard Clinical Research Institute, Harvard
Medical School, Boston, Massachusetts

DAVID A. ZIDAR, MD, PhD
Associate Professor, Department of
Cardiology, Harrington Heart and Vascular
Institute, University Hospitals Case Medical
Center, Case Western Reserve University
School of Medicine, Cleveland, Ohio

CONTENTS

The history of coronary angioplasty began with the groundbreaking work of Andreas Grüntzig, who was the first to use balloon-expandable catheters for the treatment of flow-limiting atherosclerotic coronary artery lesions. Thereafter, early investigators tested self-expanding springs as a solution to abrupt closure and restenosis seen with balloon angioplasty but these devices suffered from difficult delivery and a high complication rate. Julio Palmaz and Richard Schatz introduced the first balloon-expandable stent as a mechanical support to improve vessel patency. Their pioneering work launched a new era in the treatment of coronary artery disease.

Restenosis is a pathologic response to vascular injury, characterized by neointimal hyperplasia and progressive narrowing of a stented vessel segment. Although advances in stent design have led to a dramatic reduction in the incidence of restenosis, it continues to represent the most common cause of target lesion failure following percutaneous coronary intervention. Efforts to maximize restenosis prevention, through careful consideration of modifiable risk factors and an individualized approach, are critical, as restenosis, once established, can be particularly difficult to treat. Novel approaches are on the horizon that have the potential to alter the natural history of this stubborn disease.

The coronary stent has propelled our understanding of the term "biocompatibility." Stents are expanded at sites of arterial blockage and mechanically reestablish blood flow. This simplicity belies the complex reactions that occur when a stent contacts living substrates. Biocompatible seek to elicit the intended response; stents should perform rather than merely exist. Because performance is assessed in the patient, stent biocompatibility is the multiscale examination of material and cell, and of material, structure, and device in the context of cell, tissue, and organism. This review tracks major biomaterial advances in coronary stent design and discusses biocompatibility clinical performance.

Endovascular drug delivery continues to revolutionize the treatment of athero-sclerosis in coronary and peripheral vasculature. The key has been to identify biologic agents that can counter the hyperplastic tissue responses to device expansion/implantation and to develop effective local delivery strategies that can maintain efficacious drug levels across the artery wall over the course of de-vice effects. This article reviews the evolution of endovascular drug delivery technology, explains the mechanisms they use for drug release, and provides a quantitative mechanistic framework for relating drug release mode to arterial drug distribution and effect.

Cardiovascular disease is a leading cause of death and disability worldwide. Current treatment strategies aimed at treating the symptoms and conse-quences of obstructive vascular disease have embraced both optimal medical therapy and catheter-based percutaneous coronary intervention with drug-eluting stents. Drug-eluting stents elute antiproliferative drugs inhibiting vascular smooth muscle cell proliferation, which occurs in response to injury and thus prevents restenosis. However, all drugs currently approved for use in drug-eluting stents do not discriminate between proliferating vascular smooth muscle cells and endothelial cells, thus delaying re-endothelialization and subsequent vascular healing.

First-generation drug-eluting stents significantly improved treatment of coro-nary disease, decreasing rates of revascularization. This was offset by high rates of late adverse events, driven primarily by stent thrombosis. Research and design improvements of individual DES platform components led to next-generation devices with superior clinical safety and efficacy profiles compared with bare-metal stents and first-generation drug-eluting stents. These design improvements and features are explored, and their resulting clinical safety and efficacy reviewed, focusing on platforms approved by the Food and Drug Administration currently widely used in the United States.

The concept for a bioresorbable vascular scaffold combines the best features of the first 3 generations of percutaneous coronary intervention (namely), balloon angioplasty, bare metallic stents, and drug-eluting stents, into a single device. The principles of operation of a BRS follow 3 phases of functionality that reflect the different physiologic requirements over time; revascularization, restoration, and resorption. Most BRS designs make use of the continuum of hydrolytic degradation in aliphatic polyesters, such as poly(L-lactide), in which molecular weight, strength, and mass decrease progressively in 3 distinct stages, consistent with the in vivo requirements of each performance phase.

Bioresorbable scaffolds (BRS) have been engineered to eliminate the theoretic stimulus to late coronary events, a caveat of conventional metallic drug-eluting stents (DESs). Outcome benefits of BRSs over current-generation DESs are expected to accrue after complete bioresorption. Before this timeframe, BRSs need to prove at least similarly safe and effective compared with DESs. Several randomized studies of the Absorb BRS have been made available. Several manufacturers are at the beginning of their line of clinical development of competing BRSs. This article reviews the contemporary clinical outcomes of the Absorb scaffold, and provides an updated state of the art on the other players in the BRS arena.

Endovascular stenting has evolved over the last 50 years since its inception into the framework of management of vascular atherosclerotic disease. Stent design has evolved as lesion complexity has increased. Nevertheless, certain first principles regarding stent design have been recapitulated time and again with every iteration of endovascular stents. This article reviews principles of endovascular stent design and compares and contrasts key aspects of balloon expandable and self-expanding stents.

Endovascular treatment for aortic abnormality is an excellent alternative option for patients who are not good candidates for conventional open surgery. Although the technique of placing endovascular stent grafts has evolved since the first grafts, the basic principles remain the same. Use of endografts is limited by anatomic criteria, and advances in graft design have allowed for more widespread use for a broader patient range. The most important limitations to overcome are achieving high-quality aortic neck "healthy" landing zone, smaller-diameter delivery systems, and endografts that allow for more angled aortic necks.

Contemporary endovascular stents are the product of an iterative design and development process that leverages evolving concepts in vascular biology and engineering. This article reviews how insights into vascular pathophysiology, materials science, and design mechanics drive stent design and explain modes of stent failure. Current knowledge of pathologic processes is providing a more complete picture of the factors mediating stent failure. Further evolution of endovascular stents includes bioresorbable platforms tailored to treat plaques acutely and to then disappear after lesion pacification. Ongoing refinement of stent technology will continue to require insights from pathology to understand adverse events, refine clinical protocols, and drive innovation.

Coronary Stent Failure: Fracture, Compression, Recoil, and Prolapse   **405**
Dominik M. Wiktor, Stephen W. Waldo, and Ehrin J. Armstrong

Current-generation coronary drug-eluting stents are associated with low rates of restenosis and target lesion revascularization. However, several mechanisms of stent failure remain clinically important. Stent fracture may occur in areas of excessive torsion or angulation. Longitudinal stent deformation is related to axial stent compression owing to extrinsic forces or secondary devices that disrupt stent architecture. Stent recoil occurs when a stent does not deploy at its optimal cross-sectional area. Tissue prolapse between stent struts may also predispose patients to adverse outcomes. Prevention, recognition, and treatment of these stent failures are necessary to optimize patient outcomes after percutaneous coronary interventions.

CORONARY AND ENDOVASCULAR STENTS

THE CLINICS ARE NOW AVAILABLE ONLINE!

Access your subscription at:
www.theclinics.com

CORONARY AND ENDOVASCULAR STENTS

FORTHCOMING ISSUES

October 2016
Controversies in the Management of STEMI
Timothy Henry, Editor

January 2017
Antiplatelet and Anticoagulation Therapy
in PCI
Dominick Angiolillo and Matthew Price,
Editors

RECENT ISSUES

April 2016
Complex Coronary Intervention
Michael Lee, Editor

January 2016
Transcatheter Mitral Valve Intervention
Jason Rogers, Editor

ISSUE OF RELATED INTEREST

Heart Failure Clinics, April 2015 (Vol. 11, No. 2)
Interventional and Device Therapy in Heart Failure
Deepak L. Bhatt and Michael R. Gold, Editors
Available at: http://www.heartfailure.theclinics.com/

PREFACE

Stent Design: Past, Present, and Future

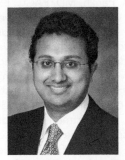

Sahil A. Parikh, MD, FACC, FSCAI
Editor

Endovascular stents have revolutionized the treatment of atherosclerotic vascular disease. However, from an engineering perspective, the advent of the stent did not immediately herald a tectonic shift in clinical practice. Rather, the endovascular stent exemplifies the marriage between engineering and empiric clinical research, a union that matures slowly. Over four decades, clinicians and patients, vascular biologists and clinical investigators, engineers and entrepreneurs collaborated closely to deliver the coronary drug-eluting stent, arguably one of the greatest breakthroughs in cardiovascular medicine in the past half century. Important lessons learned from the coronary experience have translated into novel applications of stents in other vascular beds. In this compendium, it was our intention to highlight some of the critical facets of stent design that serve as the foundation for endovascular interventions throughout the circulation.

Our journey through stent design begins with a historical perspective from Dr Richard Schatz, who offers his first-hand view of the development of one of the first coronary stents. This is followed by Dr David Zidar's comprehensive review of restenosis biology, which underpins the rationale for the development of endovascular stents. The next several articles focus on the critical biomedical engineering principles that underlie the development of all endovascular stents: biocompatibility (Dr Kumaran Kolandaivelu) and endovascular drug delivery (Dr Abraham Tzafriri).

The first principles outlined in these two cogent reviews serve as a handbook for features that will undoubtedly underpin future evolutions in the field. Dr Aloke Finn next lends perspective to the critical importance of antiproliferative therapies in the development of drug-eluting stents to inhibit restenosis. The discussion is salient to the development of noncoronary stents as well. Dr Robert Yeh then helps summarize the data supporting coronary drug-eluting stents, the dominant mode of coronary revascularization in the developed world.

Subsequently, our focus shifts to review novel technologies that represent strategic adaptations of fundamental stent design principles. These include bioresorbable scaffolds reviewed by Dr Richard Rapoza and Dr Davide Cappodanno as well as adaptations from small- and medium-sized vessels to large vessels such as those encountered in the peripheral vasculature and aorta reviewed by me and Dr Vikram Kashyap, respectively. I would highlight that the fundamental first principles of small-vessel stent design underlie all of these novel adaptations. Finally, the issue concludes with reviews of stent pathology (Dr Abraham Tzafriri) and stent complications (Dr Ehrin Armstrong).

The articles in this issue of *Interventional Cardiology Clinics* serve as a succinct review of the state of the art in endovascular stent design. The articles are written with the clinician in mind to better inform practitioners in the science that

Intervent Cardiol Clin 5 (2016) xi–xii
http://dx.doi.org/10.1016/j.iccl.2016.05.001
2211-7458/16/$ – see front matter © 2016 Published by Elsevier Inc.

rests behind the devices we use every day. We believe that the principles outlined in this issue will remain salient even as the field races forward. We expect that clinical trainees and experienced practitioners alike will find value in these collected works.

I would be remiss if I did not thank all of the authors in this issue for their expertise, time, and patience. We have assembled experts from a diverse array of fields that subsume many of the key stakeholders in the field of stent design, including clinician scientists, biomedical engineers, academic investigators, and industry representatives. Importantly, this issue would not have been possible without the support of Dr Matthew Price, the Consulting Editor of *Interventional Cardiology Clinics*, and the entire staff at Elsevier, especially Lauren Boyle, Adrianne Brigido, and Susan Showalter. Finally, I wish to thank my scientific mentor, Dr Elazer Reuven Edelman, whose indelible imprint on the field of endovascular stents and my own career has been profound and everlasting.

Sahil A. Parikh, MD, FACC, FSCAI
Case Western Reserve University
School of Medicine
Center for Research and Innovation
Interventional Cardiology Fellowship Program
University Hospitals Harrington
Heart and Vascular Institute
Division of Cardiovascular Medicine
Department of Medicine
University Hospitals Case Medical Center
11100 Euclid Avenue
Cleveland, OH 44106, USA
E-mail address:
Sahil.Parikh@UHhospitals.org

The History of Coronary Stenting

Christina Tan, MD, Richard A. Schatz, MD*

KEYWORDS

- Coronary stents • Palmaz-Schatz stent • Coronary angioplasty • Interventional cardiology

KEY POINTS

- Angioplasty results were limited by abrupt closure and restenosis, leading investigation into self-expanding metal coils in experimental models.
- Dr Julio Palmaz conceived of the first balloon-expandable slotted tube concept stainless steel stent in the late 1970s.
- Palmaz and Dr Richard Schatz placed the first stents in dog coronaries in 1985 and the first humans in 1987.
- Drug-coated stents and new antiplatelet agents significantly reduced rates of in-stent restenosis and stent thrombosis, respectively.
- With ever-improving designs and drug release platforms, stents are now the cornerstone of interventional therapy for treating coronary artery disease worldwide.

INTRODUCTION

There is no discipline in the history of medicine that has seen an explosion of growth and innovation like that of interventional cardiology, due to a combination of a driving need for better results in the treatment of coronary artery disease and the unique personality of individuals drawn to the field. In the early 1970s, the treatment of coronary disease was limited to nitroglycerin and propranolol, few diagnostic tests, no randomized trials, and little understanding of the acute phases of myocardial infarction. Diagnostic angiography was a new procedure, with crude equipment by today's standards.

Bypass surgery was an exciting new option but strictly reserved for patients who had severe angina despite maximal medical therapy. Angiography was strongly discouraged unless a patient had refractory symptoms and a very positive stress test. Noninvasive testing did not exist as it is known today and not until the late 1970s did echocardiography and nuclear medicine become widely available as adjuncts to the basic treadmill.

The treatment of myocardial infarction was even more rudimentary by today's standards. Patients were admitted to an intensive care unit and given oxygen and morphine only, while furosemide and aminophylline were added if the patient developed symptoms of congestive heart failure. It was not unusual for a patient to be hospitalized for 4 to 6 weeks during the observation period. Much consternation and anxiety was generated for both patient and physician during this period.

The entire world changed in September 1977, when a daring young doctor from Basel, Switzerland, performed the first angioplasty on a conscious patient with a tight lesion of the left anterior descending artery. Dr Andreas Grüntzig had been quietly working on a concept that he conceived while studying under one of the great mentors of the time, Dr Charles Dotter. Grüntzig had watched Dotter's procedure of dilating peripheral arterial stenoses with tapered tubes and conceived the idea of adding a balloon to the tip and a central lumen inside the catheter to fill the balloon with contrast material. On expansion of the balloon at the target site, the

No conflicts of interest or financial disclosures.
Division of Cardiology, Scripps Clinic, 10666 North Torrey Pines Road, La Jolla, CA 92037, USA
* Corresponding author.
E-mail address: schatz.richard@scrippshealth.org

Intervent Cardiol Clin 5 (2016) 271–280
http://dx.doi.org/10.1016/j.iccl.2016.03.001

plaque would give way (like crushed snow) and hopefully remain open. He was able to build a catheter suitable for human use and after much difficulty got permission to try the first case in a human. Fortunately, the case could not have gone better and the patient walked out of the hospital angina-free without bypass surgery. The world would never be the same.[1]

Grüntzig's work spread like wildfire around the world. Eventually, after meeting resistance at home, Grüntzig moved to the United States in 1980 and built the stage for teaching his new procedure at Emory University, soon to become the world center for this new discipline, interventional cardiology. Thousands of doctors made the pilgrimage to Emory to learn the technique and then return home to start their own programs. Grüntzig was meticulous and painfully honest at collecting data on his new procedure and encouraged registries, randomized trials, and collaboration to understand the limitations of what he was proposing. Unfortunately, not all cases went smoothly, and abrupt closure, dissection, and cardiac arrest were not uncommon. At least once or twice during the demonstrations, patients would arrest and be whisked off to the waiting operating room with a young doctor straddled on top of the patient doing CPR.

Although those in Gruntzig's audience often prayed for a successful surgical save while witnessing these crashes, one observer in particular, Dr Julio Palmaz, saw it as an opportunity to improve on angioplasty technique. After seeing Grüntzig's presentation in 1977, he quickly developed the concept of a metal sleeve that could be placed on top of the balloon, carried to the site, and then deployed by balloon expansion to support the walls of the artery, preventing mechanical collapse. Surprisingly, this concept was not new because several investigators had the same idea and published widely on the topic in the 1960s.[2–6] Palmaz noted that the devices were all some variation of a self-expanding spring or coil, thus limited by imprecise expansion and unpredictable delivery, both of which could be solved with a balloon-expandable piece of metal. The challenge then became which design and which metal.

He visited RadioShack, returning with a bag full of wire, solder, and a soldering gun. Converting his kitchen table into a laboratory, Palmaz set out to build his own prototype (Fig. 1). From 1980 to 1985, Palmaz placed dozens of these "grafts" (he did not call them stents) in countless dog arteries successfully.[7] His meticulous attention to study design assured a methodical assessment of the graft tissue interaction with careful long-term follow-up and pathology (thanks to

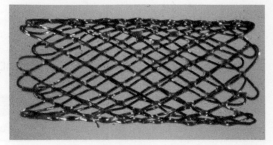

Fig. 1. The first balloon-expandable stent. This was made of 316L wire wrapped around a mandrel. Each cross-point was soldered with silver solder to prevent sliding of the wires against each other.

Dr Fermin Tio) to make sure the device was biocompatible and not toxic to the animal. Due to the size of the device, he was restricted to large straight vessels, such as iliac arteries and the descending aorta. It worked well in these areas but the real challenge was in the coronary arteries, where the risks of clotting and restenosis were amplified due to their small size.

By 1983, Palmaz moved to the University of Texas at San Antonio with his mentor Dr Stewart Reuter. He presented the data for the first time at the Radiological Society of North America in 1984 and published his first article in 1985.

With some funding from the University of Texas, Palmaz set out to accelerate his efforts. After discussion with several experts in thin metals, he soon found the right metal and the right technology. His first prototypes were made of 316L stainless steel, a common metal used for sutures and needles that already had a track record with the Food and Drug Administration (FDA) for human use. He soon replaced the wire stents with the slotted tube concept (Fig. 2). By heating the grafts he was able to

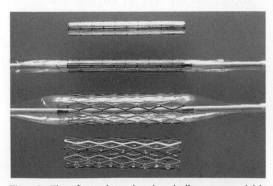

Fig. 2. The first slotted tube balloon-expandable stent. This measured 3 mm in diameter and 30 mm in length. It was cut from a hollow tube using electromagnetic discharge. It could be expanded to as much as 18 mm in diameter.

take the spring out of the metal, so, once expanded, the tube resisted recoil.

The first devices proved much easier to deliver than the originals due to their lower profile. Their size (30 mm × 3 mm) and rigid configuration made them suitable only for large straight vessels. Nonetheless, the technology was easily transferrable to smaller tubes and by 1985 Palmaz produced a prototype (Fig. 3) (15 mm × 1.5 mm), which could be placed in vessels as small as 2.5 mm and as large as 5 mm. When Dr Schatz met Palmaz in 1985, he was ready to test these grafts in coronary arteries.

Working as a team with new private funding, the pace of work increased dramatically. Within months, Schatz and Palmaz had placed scores of grafts into rabbit iliac arteries, dog coronaries, and pig renal arteries. The results confirmed that delivery was possible in smaller, straight arteries. If the animals were pretreated with a cocktail of aspirin, dipyridamole, and dextran, clotting did not occur. A randomized trial in dogs showed that this combination was essential to prevent thrombosis.[8] Even though we never saw a case of stent thrombosis in animals, we recognized that these were normal arteries and that greater challenges lay in treating diseased human vessels.

Early on Palmaz and Schatz recognized the need for a more flexible device. It was clear that the slotted tube would not be able to go through standard coronary guides, much less down human coronaries. In Europe, unbeknownst to American investigators, several investigators were working on a springlike device (Wallstent, Medivent, Lausanne, Switzerland.) with some early success[9] (Fig. 4). Much to our surprise, in March of 1986, Schatz and Palmaz got word of the first patients treated for abrupt closure long before they were ready to do their first cases. Puel, Marco, and Sigwart placed

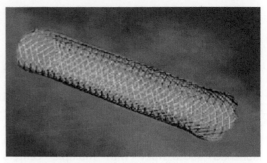

Fig. 4. The Wallstent. This was the first self-expanding stent ever used in humans. (Boston Scientific, Marlborough, MA.)

Wallstents in 2 patients with excellent results.[10] Soon after that, after abandoning a springlike device that he worked on with Grüntzig , a radiologist named Dr Cesare Gianturco developed a balloon-expandable wire coil (Fig. 5) and filed an abrupt closure trial with the FDA that required the patient to go to bypass surgery after the stent was placed. Dr Gary Roubin placed one of these coils successfully in a patient for abrupt closure at Emory University in September 1986, and the race was on!

In August 1986, Palmaz and Schatz had signed a licensing agreement with Johnson & Johnson (New Brunswick, New Jersey) and were working diligently on the iliac protocol. They had completed the first 30 dog coronary implants plus a large series of renal implants, all successful, so it was thought the coronary investigative device exemption would be easy. Much to their surprise, the PDA decided that Schatz and Palmaz should complete a peripheral trial before they could start the coronaries. The earliest discussions with the FDA from 1985 had indicated only 75 cases in the coronaries prior to submission of pre-market approval. Schatz and Palmaz also believed they had been specifically told patients would not have to be

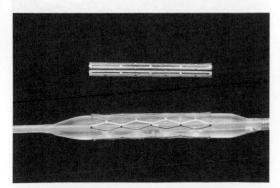

Fig. 3. This smaller version of the slotted tube stent was designed for vessels in the range of 2.5 mm to 5 mm in diameter. It was 1.5 mm in diameter and 15 mm in length.

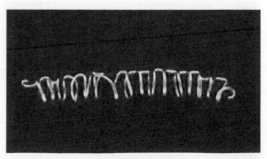

Fig. 5. The Gianturco-Roubin stent. This was the first stent placed in humans in the United States. It was made of round wire wrapped around a balloon. (Cook Medical, Bloomington, IN.)

randomized in the study, unheard of by today's standards. Furthermore, no other stent trials required a peripheral trial first.

In May 1987, Palmaz traveled to Freiburg, Germany, and placed the first iliac stent in a human along with Dr Goetz Richter. The procedure went well and it was a relief to have performed the first successful human case. Months later, they finally received FDA approval to begin the iliac trial in the United States and the trial launched successfully with multiple centers across the country. The trial was completed quickly and led to FDA approval in 1991.

It was clear that the rigid 15-mm stent would not go through the usual guiding catheters, so patients had to be selected wisely to ensure success. Therefore, the protocol was written to include only short, focal lesions in large, straight right coronary arteries with good collaterals and good left ventricular function. I wanted to make sure that if, in the worst case, the stent clotted, it would have minimal clinical impact on the patient. Furthermore, I selected the straightest catheter possible to avoid any issues with curves, either the 8-French multipurpose or 8.3-French Stertzer catheter from the right brachial cut-down approach.

It did not take long to find the first patient. Dr Eduardo D'Souza, a prolific cardiologist from São Paulo, Brazil, sent a film belonging to a young man with classic angina and a tight lesion of a down-going right coronary artery with good collaterals and normal left ventricular function. Schatz approved the case, and they set sail for Brazil in December 1987. The entourage consisted of Schatz, Palmaz, several people from Johnson & Johnson, engineers and clinical specialists from Johnson and Johnson (Fig. 6).

Things could not have gone better, until the first picture was taken. Much to Schatz's chargin, they found a total occlusion, a clot no doubt, but without an infarct, so it was presumed to have closed silently without incident due to his brisk collaterals.

They had not seen thrombosis in any of the animals which were pretreated with antiplatelets. Grüntzig had insisted on aspirin, dipyridamole, Anturane, dextran, and warfarin in all patients for fear of thrombosis. Warfarin and dextran were later eliminated. Schatz did not want to force warfarin on all patients for fear that we would not be able to stop it without a large trial. The animal work clearly showed benefit for dextran (Fig. 7). Schatz and Palmaz ballooned the lesion and got a good result without further clot, then placed a 3.0-mm stent, and then over-dilated it with a 3.5-mm balloon. The final result was excellent. The patient had an uneventful night and the next morning's follow-up angiogram showed a widely patent stent. He was discharged that day on aspirin and dipyridamole without warfarin and remained asymptomatic for many years. His several follow-up angiograms showed only mild intimal hyperplasia (Fig. 8).

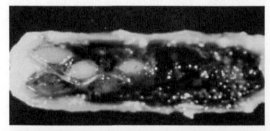

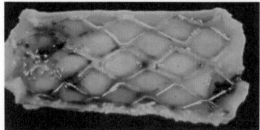

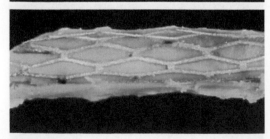

Fig. 7. Three stents from dogs treated with different anticoagulation regimens. The top stent came from a dog, which did not receive any medication prior to placement. The middle stent was from a dog treated with aspirin, heparin, and dipyridamole. The bottom stent shows the difference when dextran was added in addition to aspirin, heparin, and dipyridamole.

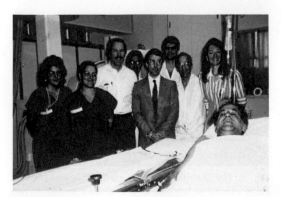

Fig. 6. The São Paulo, Brazil, team and the first patient to receive a Palmaz coronary stent.

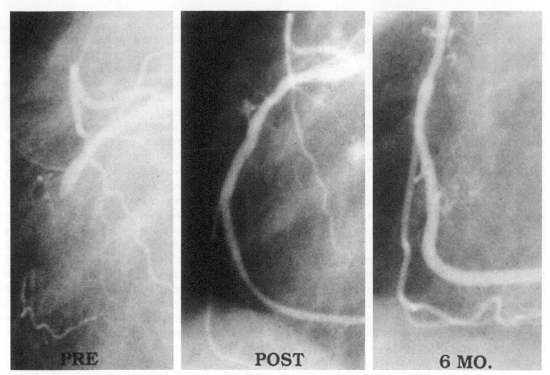

Fig. 8. The first rigid stent ever placed in a human coronary artery. The left panel is pre, the middle panel is post, and the right panel is 6 months. There was moderate intimal hyperplasia by IVUS at follow-up. The patient remained asymptomatic for 13 years.

After this success, Palmaz and Schatz visited many other sites around the world to introduce the procedure to anyone who would listen. They were also working on a more flexible version, which consisted of two or three 7-mm slotted tube segments connected with a short flexible strut (**Fig. 9**). The animal testing went better than expected proving that this articulated version could navigate through all conventional guides and into all the coronaries. The stents still required hand crimping, which made all of us nervous because the balloons available were low profile and slippery, the exact opposite of what was needed.

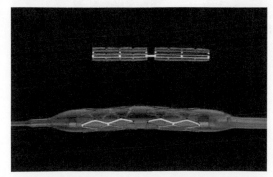

Fig. 9. The first articulated PSS. (Cordis Corporation, Hialeah, FL.)

Worldwide, both the Wallstent and Gianturco-Roubin stents were concurrently gaining traction because they were more flexible and easier to deliver than the Palmaz-Schatz stent (PSS). This proved a nagging setback for quite some time.

In spite of the delay of iliac investigative device exemption approval, the coronary protocol was approved in 8 weeks. Finally, Schatz and Palmaz were ready to do their first cases in the United States by January 1988, using the rigid prototype. The first case in February 1988 at the Arizona Heart Institute in Phoenix went terribly wrong because the stent could not be delivered due to tortuosity in the vessel. The stent would not pass the lesion and there was the potential to lose the stent entirely without possibility of retrieval, so Schatz chose to deply it proximal to the target lesion. The patient later underwent bypass surgery for restenosis. This was another wake up call that the flexible stent should be released as soon as possible.

In May 1988, Schatz and Palmaz received permission from Johnson & Johnson to place the first articulated stent, the PSS, in humans. They set out to Mainz, Germany, where a single PSS was placed in a patient's proximal left anterior descending coronary artery with Dr Raimund Erbel. The procedure was a great success and proved that the new design was flexible enough to go through a Judkins curve and down the left anterior descending coronary artery (**Fig. 10**).[11]

The rest of the year, Palmaz and Schatz opened new centers all over the world with the flexible stent. Despite optimistic early results, reports of stent embolization, thrombosis, and major bleeding became more and more prevalent. With the coronary protocol in the United States, similar concerns were being voiced. Although subacute stent thrombosis (SAT) did not occur in the first 10 to 15 patients, this serious complication spiked to almost 2.8% once the protocol was opened to the new centers.[12] It was also noted that unlike angioplasty, acute early thrombosis (<24 hours) did not occur.

By December of 1988, as a result of growing concern from investigators, Johnson & Johnson (now Johnson & Johnson Interventional Systems) decided to recommend warfarin in all patients receiving a coronary stent in addition to aspirin and dipyridamole. After reviewing many of the SAT cases, Schatz thought that the cause for SAT was more operator error and incomplete expansion of the stent than not enough anticoagulation. It was only years later when Columbo and colleagues[13] reconfirmed the importance

of full stent expansion along with the introduction of newer antiplatelet agents, such as ticlopidine, that SAT dropped from approximately 5% to a more acceptable 1% to 2% without warfarin. As predicted, however, bleeding complications increased from adding warfarin, usually from groin hematomas.[14]

In 1987, Sigwart and colleagues[10] published the first article summarizing preclinical and clinical results with the Wallstent, showing encouraging early nonrandomized results. Without regulatory barriers, all 3 available stents were being sold and used widely outside the United States, although there were few but anecdotal data published.[15–19] In general it was agreed that both the Wallstent and the Gianturco-Roubin stent were more flexible, thus more deliverable, than the PSS; however, they all suffered from SAT and restenosis. Embolization was a serious problem with both the Gianturco-Roubin and PSS.

The first solution to solve the flexibility problem was to construct a subselective sheath system (**Fig. 11**) to protect the stent from wall contact. This worked reasonably well but was still difficult to deliver to tortuous or distal parts of the vessel. Eventually, a custom sheath system was developed by PAS Systems, San Francisco,

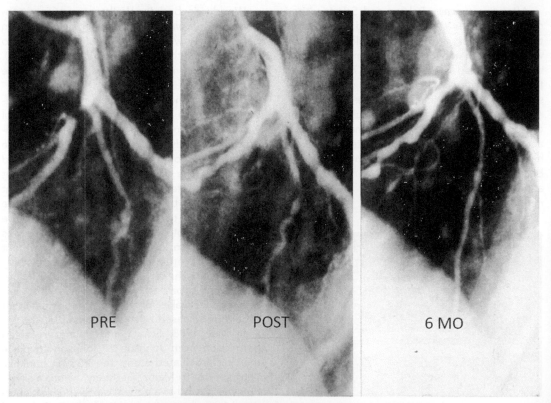

PRE   POST   6 MO

Fig. 10. The first PSS placed in the proximal left anterior descending artery in a patient in Mainz, Germany. The left panel is pre, the middle panel is post, and the right panel is 6 months' follow-up.

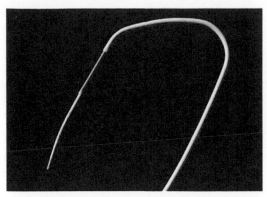

Fig. 11. Our first attempt to prevent stent embolization. This was a 5-French custom guiding catheter inside a 7-French guiding catheter, which was placed across the target lesion first. The stent was then advanced inside the 5-French sheath until it was past the lesion after which the sheath was withdrawn.

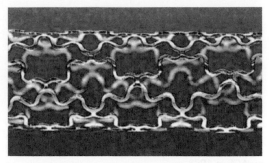

Fig. 13. The Crown stent. This modification of the PSS incorporated a wavy design in the metal struts to improve flexibility.

California, dubbed the Stent Delivery System (Fig. 12). This was provided for all US investigators as well and eventually released with FDA approval. Although an overall improvement, delivery was difficult due to the bulky size of the outer sheath. It was not until years later when Johnson & Johnson Interventional Systems, now Cordis Corporation (Lakewood, Florida), developed the Crown stent with a nesting technique that secured the stent to the balloon well enough such that the sheath could be eliminated (Fig. 13). Later, the PSS evolved into another stent called the Velocity (Fig. 14), also a slotted tube but with an S-shaped connector instead of a straight connector between the slots. This further improved flexibility and later became

the platform for the first drug-coated stent, Cypher, Johnson & Johnson Interventional Systems, Warren, New Jersey.

Embolization was not as common with the Wallstent; however, its widespread use was hampered by both stent thrombosis and restenosis.[10,20] Two complications proved fatal to the success of both the Wallstent and Gianturco-Roubin stent and over time they gradually disappeared from the market.

Two large randomized trials were conducted, in the United States (STRESS, n = 410) and in Europe (BENESTENT, n = 520); both were designed to test whether coronary stenting reduced restenosis compared with balloon angioplasty in de novo single native coronary lesions. Much was riding on the outcome of these 2 studies. Fortunately, both demonstrated similar outcomes with a significant reduction in restenosis in the stent group compared with angioplasty (42% vs 31% for STRESS, P<.046, and 32% vs 22%, P<.02, for BENESTENT).[21,22] Although the FDA rejected the PSS in 1993 initially, they later approved it in the United States in 1994 and, once approved, sales took off briskly both in and outside of the United States.

In 1998, Advanced Cardiac Sciences (ACS) released the Mulit-Link stent, another slotted tube design but with alternating open slots (Fig. 15). It had thinner struts and was more

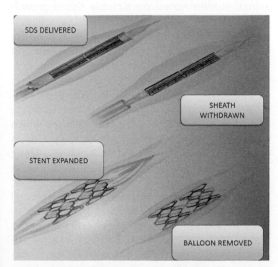

Fig. 12. The Stent Delivery System (SDS). This was the commercial version of the delivery system, which was used in the United States after FDA approval.

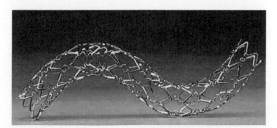

Fig. 14. The Velocity stent. A further modification of the PSS, which included an S-shaped connector between the slotted tube members instead of a straight strut.

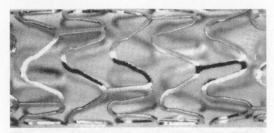

Fig. 15. The Multi-Link stent. This was the first open designed slotted tube stent developed and released by ACS in 1998.

flexible than the PSS and Crown and quickly took over the bulk of the market share. Another company, called Advanced Vascular Engineering (AVE, Santa Rosa, CA), released the Micro Stent, and later the GFX stent, another closed slotted tube design made of smooth round wire and welded connectors (Fig. 16). Again no randomized data were available comparing it to the Multi-Link or Crown; however, registry data showed it comparable. Soon both of these stents shared the bulk of the market with the Crown a distant third. ACS was soon acquired by Guidant, Indianapolis, Indiana, then Eli Lilly (Indianapolis, Indiana) and AVE by Medtronic (Minneapolis, Minnesota). Stents enjoyed enormous success once warfarin was eliminated and intravascular ultrasound (IVUS) showed the importance of full stent expansion. Along with newer antiplatelet agents, this made stents the most successful launch of medical devices in history.

Although restenosis rates for all stent designs remained approximately 15% to 20% and SAT approximately 1% for routine cases, stent use rapidly expanded far beyond its FDA indication of single de novo lesions in 3.0-mm to 3.5-mm native vessels. With no data at all, stents were being used off-label for acute myocardial infarction, saphenous vein bypass grafts, chronic total occlusions, bifurcations, long lesions, short lesions, and more. Eventually, the data caught up and revealed that restenosis rates were not

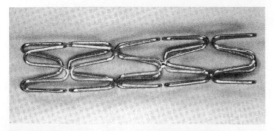

Fig. 16. The Micro stent. This slotted tube stent was released by AVE in 2000. It incorporated rounded edges of the slots instead of rectangles and a welded connector between the slotted tube members.

really 15% to 20% but higher in these more complicated patients. SAT also was higher than expected, especially in unstable patients with clot or acute myocardial infarction.[23] Design changes in the fundamental stainless steel platform had peaked so it became clear that the nagging restenosis and SAT problems would have to be solved by pharmacologic advances in surface coating and drug delivery system.

Palmaz and I had predicted this and our earliest patents claimed the coating of the stent surface with anticoagulants, such as heparin, to prevent clotting. In the early1990s we started working with Cordis on the first heparin-coated stent and after encouraging animal work treated the first patients in approximately1995 after FDA approval. This product was released worldwide shortly thereafter and was used for the first time in a major trial, the BENESTENT II trial.[24] Resumption of heparin was progressively delayed after stenting and in the final group aspirin and ticlopidine were used instead of warfarin and heparin. There was no SAT in any of the patients and the bleeding complication rate was reduced from 7.9% to 0 in the final group. This study demonstrated that heparin coating reduced both SAT and bleeding complications. We now needed to address restenosis as well with a pharmacologic approach to reduce intimal hyperplasia. Without a substantial reduction in restenosis, coronary artery bypass graft would remain a superior strategy for complex multivessel coronary disease.

Restenosis was long understood to be the result of exuberant smooth muscle tissue growth inside the stent. The earliest publications from animal studies noted predictable tissue growth inside the stent at various intervals of sampling.[25] Early thick cellular proliferation at 4 to 8 weeks gave way to an acellular matrix by 32 weeks and longer. Isner and others confirmed that the predominant cause of in-stent restenosis was smooth muscle cell proliferation.[26] Once the molecular pathways were understood, various drugs targeting the cell cycle were tested to see which were most suitable for a stent coating. Cordis developed the first such system by using a static cell inhibitor, rapamycin (sirolimus). By acting at the target of rapamycin receptor of the cell cycle, cellular proliferation was interrupted to limit cell growth, thus reducing restenosis. The first human trials were exciting, showing no restenosis in the first patients treated (REALITY trial[27]). Larger trials followed, showing an impressively low restenosis rate of 5% to 7% in benign de novo lesions of native coronary arteries. This new stent, Cypher, Johnson & Johnson Interventional

Systems, Warren, New Jersey, was launched in 2003 on a new slotted tube platform called Velocity, designed to be more flexible than the earlier Crown and PSS stents.

Soon after, in 2005, Boston Scientific launched Taxol, a commonly used cytotoxic cancer drug, as a stent coating on their NIR, then Liberté, slotted tube platform, now called the Taxus stent. Early data showed impressive reduction in restenosis rates below 10% despite a higher late loss than Cypher.[28]

As more data became available, it became clear that a new phenomenon of late and very late thrombosis was evolving. Autopsy data from Vermani and colleagues[29] showed a clear inflammatory reaction in patients with late SAT thought to result directly from the polymer barriers used to control release of the drug into the circulation. This prompted development of more powerful antiplatelet agents and longer duration of treatment up to 1 year or longer.

In 2008, Medtronic released the first nonpolymer, phospholipid-based coating on their Zotarolimus drug-eluting stent Endeavor, designed to be more biologically compatible than previous polymers. Although SAT was not lowered substantially, a shorter requirement for antiplatelet agents was suggested in at least 1 study (SENS trial[30]). Animal and human studies suggested a more functional endothelium with Endeavor compared with Cypher and Taxus,[31] responding to acetylcholine with more vasodilation than vasoconstriction.

In 2009, Abbott, California and Boston Scientific released the latest product in the stent world, the Xience/Promus stent using everolimus and a unique coating for delivery. The new stents showed similar results to all prior stents with restenosis rates below 10% and SAT rates of 1% to 2%.[32] The only true randomized trial comparing 3 of the stents (Cypher, Taxus, and Endeavor), the ZEST trial, showed no advantage to any one of them over the others at 3 years of follow-up.[33]

The newest breakthroughs in stent technology include bioabsorbable stents, cobalt chromium platforms, absorbable polymers, and nanotechnology surface treatments to avoid polymer coatings, all of which will hopefully solve the elusive problems of stent thrombosis and restenosis.

There is no way we could have foreseen the impact of our work so many years ago. Some 28 years after the first stents were placed in humans, the basic balloon-expandable slotted tube metal platform has stood the test of time and remains the fundamental cornerstone of modern-day therapy for the treatment of coronary artery disease. The mechanical contribution to restenosis and abrupt closure has been solved, making emergency bypass surgery a thing of the past. Now the challenge is to develop the right cocktail of drugs and coatings to eliminate, not just reduce, thrombosis and restenosis entirely. Stents have taken Grüntzig's dream of repairing coronary arteries in the conscious human patient to the next level and have allowed creating dreams of 1 day eliminating bypass surgery completely. With the precedent set of designing vigorous randomized trials and constantly questioning the status quo, I believe we will see this in our lifetime. Were Grüntzig alive today, we think he would be very proud of what we have accomplished.

REFERENCES

1. Gruentzig AR, Senning A, Siegenthaler WE. Nonoperative dilatation of coronary-artery stenosis: percutaneous transluminal coronary angioplasty. N Engl J Med 1979;301:61–8.
2. Dotter CT. Transluminally placed coil-spring endarterial tubegrafts, long-term patency in canine popliteal artery. Invest Radiol 1969;4:329–32.
3. Dotter CT, Buschmann RW, McKinney MK, et al. Transluminal expandable nitinol coil stent grafting: preliminary report. Radiology 1983;147:259–60.
4. Cragg A, Lund G, Rysavy J, et al. Nonsurgical placement of arterial endoprosthesis: a new technique using nitinol wire. Radiology 1983;147:261–3.
5. Cragg A, Lung G, Rysavy JA, et al. Percutaneous arterial grafting. Radiology 1984;150:45–9.
6. Maass D, Zollikofer CL, Largiader F, et al. Radiological follow-up of transluminally inserted endoprostheses: an experimental study using expandable spirals. Radiology 1984;152:659–63.
7. Palmaz JC, Sibbitt RR, Reuter SR, et al. Expandable intraluminal graft: a preliminary study. Work in progress. Radiology 1985;156(1):73–7.
8. Palmaz JC, Garcia O, Kopp DB, et al. Balloon-expandable intra-arterial stents: effect of antithrombotic medication on thrombus formation. In: Seither C, Seyferth W, editors. Pros and Cons in PTA and auxillary methods. Berlin: Springer-Verlag; 1989.
9. Rousseau H, Puel J, Joffre F, et al. Self-expanding endovascular prosthesis: an experimential study. Radiology 1987;164:709–14.
10. Sigwart U, Puel J, Mirkovitch V, et al. Intravascular stents to prevent occlusion and restenosis after transluminal angioplasty. N Engl J Med 1987;316:701–6.
11. Schatz RA, Palmaz JC, Tio F, et al. Report of a new articulated balloon expandable intravascular stent [abstract]. Circulation 1988;78(Suppl II):449.

12. Schatz RA, Goldberg S, Leon M, et al. Clinical experience with the Palmaz-Schatz coronary stent. J Am Coll Cardiol 1991;17(6):155B–9B.

13. Columbo A, Hall P, Nakamura S, et al. Intracoronary stenting without anticoagulation accomplished with intravascular ultrasound guidance. Circulation 1995;91:1676.

14. Schatz RA, Baim DS, Leon M, et al. Clinical experience with the Palmaz-Schatz coronary stent: initial results of a multicenter study. Circulation 1991;83:148–61.

15. Roubin GS, Douglas JS, Lembo NJ, et al. Intracoronary stenting for acute closure following percutaenous trasnluminal coronary angioplasty (PTCA) [abstract]. Circulation 1988;78(Suppl II):II-407.

16. Sigwart U, Urban P, Gold S, et al. Emergency stenting for acute occlusion after coronary balloon angioplasty. Circulation 1988;79:1121–7.

17. Urban P, Sigwart U, Gold S, et al. Intravascular stenting for stenosis of aortocoronary venous bypass grafts. J Am Coll Cardiol 1989;13:1085–91.

18. Sigwart U, Urban P, Sadeghi H, et al. Implantation of 100 coronary artery stents: learning curve for the incidence of acute early complications [abstract]. J Am Coll Cardiol 1989;13:107A.

19. Sigwart U, Gold S, Kaufman U, et al. Analysis of complications associated with coronary stenting [abstract]. L Am Coll Cardiol 1988;11:66A.

20. Lansky AJ, Roubin GS, O'Shaughnessy CD, et al. Randomized comparison of GR-II stent and Palmaz-Schatz stent for elective treatment of coronary stenoses. Circulation 2000;102:1364–8.

21. Fischman DL, Leon M, Baim DS, et al. A randomized comparison of coronary stent placement and balloon angioplasty in the treatment of coronary artery disease. N Engl J Med 1994;27:255–61.

22. Serruys PW, de Jaegere P, Kiemeneij F, et al, For the Benestent Study Group. A comparison of balloon-expandable stent implantation with balloon angioplasty in patients with coronary artery disease. N Engl J Med 1994;331:489–95.

23. Grines CL. Off-label use of drug-eluting stents putting it in perspective. J Am Coll Cardiol 2008;51(6):615–7.

24. Serruys PW, Emanuelsson H, van der Giessen W, et al, On behalf of the Benestent II Study Group. Heparin-coated stents in hyman coronary arteries: early outcome of Benestent II pilot study. Circulation 1996;93:412–22.

25. Schatz RA, Palmaz JC, Tio FO, et al. Balloon-expandable intracoronary stents in the adult dog. Circulation 1987;76:450–7.

26. Kearney M, Pieczek A, Isner J, et al. Histopathology of In-Stent Restenosis in Patients with Peripheral Artery Disease. Circulation 1997;95:1998–2002.

27. Morice MC, Colombo A, Meier B, et al. Sirolimus-vs paclitaxel-eluting stents in de novo coronary artery lesions. The REALITY trial: a randomized controlled trial. JAMA 2006;295:895–904.

28. Dawkins KD, Grube E, Guagliumi G, et al, On behalf of the TAXUS VI Investigators. Clinical efficacy of polymer-based paclitaxel-eluting stents in the treatment of complex, long coronary artery lesions from a multicenter, randomized trial, Support for the use of drug-eluting stents in contemporary clinical practice. Circulation 2005;112:3306–13.

29. Joner M, Virmani R. Pathology of Drug-Eluting Stents in Humans. J AM Coll Cardiol 2006;48(1):193–202.

30. Kim JW, Kang WC, Kim KS, et al. Outcome of non-surgical procedure and brief interruption of dual anti-platelet therapy in patients within 12 months following Endeavor (zotarolimus-eluting stent) stent implantation (SENS): a multicenter study. J Am Coll Cardiol 2009;53(Suppl):A16.

31. Kandzari DE, Mauri L, Popma JJ, et al. Late-term clinical outcomes with zotarolimus- and sirolimus-eluting stents. 5-year follow-up of the ENDEAVOR III (A randomized controlled trial of the Medtronic Endeavor Drug [ABT-578] leuting coronary stent system versus the Cypher sirolimus-eluting coronary stent system in de novo native coronary artery lesions). JACC Cardiovasc Interv 2011;4(5):543–50.

32. Garg S, Serruys P, Onuma Y, et al. 3-Year clinical follow-up of the XIENCE V Everolimus-eluting coronary stent system in the treatment of patients with de novo coronary artery lesions. The SPIRIT II Trial (Clinical Evaluation of the Xience V Everolimus Eluting Coronary Stent System in the Treatment of Patients with de novo Native Coronary Artery Lesions). JACC Cardiovasc Interv 2009;2(12):1190–8.

33. Park DW, Kim YH, Yun SC, et al. Comparison of Zotarolimus-Eluting Stents with Sirolimus- and Paclitaxel-Eluting Stents for Coronary Revascularization. The ZEST (Comparison of the Efficacy and Safety of Zotarolimus-Eluting Stent with Sirolimus-Eluting and PacliTaxel-Eluting Stent for Coronary Lesions) Randomized Trial. J Am Coll Cardiol 2010;56(15):1187–95.

Restenosis of the Coronary Arteries
Past, Present, Future Directions

Julius B. Elmore, MD, Emile Mehanna, MD,
Sahil A. Parikh, MD, David A. Zidar, MD, PhD*

KEYWORDS

- Restenosis • Coronary arteries • Neointimal hyperplasia • Progressive narrowing

KEY POINTS

- Restenosis, a pathologic response to injury, leads to narrowing of a stented vessel segment due to negative vascular remodeling and neointimal proliferation of vascular smooth muscle cells.
- Restenosis remains the most common cause of target lesion failure, and its predictors include diabetes, smoking status, female gender, acute coronary syndrome, previous percutaneous coronary intervention, saphenous vein graft disease, small vessel diameter, long lesions, high angiographic complexity, ostial location, and chronic total occlusions.
- The diameter achieved at the end of the procedure is an important modifiable predictor of restenosis.
- The prevention and optimal treatment of restenosis depend on several angiographic and clinical features and thus require an individualized approach.

BACKGROUND

Coronary artery restenosis, an exuberant response to mechanical injury of the arterial segment leading to lumen loss after percutaneous intervention, has plagued cardiologists since the introduction of balloon angioplasty by Gruntzig[1] and continues to do so despite contemporary drug-eluting stent (DES) technology. This article describes the mechanisms, clinical features, impact, and treatment options of restenosis after percutaneous coronary intervention (PCI).

Definition and Incidence

Obstruction of 50% or more of the diameter of a stenosis within 5 mm of a previously treated coronary segment is historically defined as binary angiographic restenosis.[2] Clinically driven restenosis rates are typically half that of binary restenosis.[3]

Late loss (LL), a continuous angiographic measure of lumen deterioration, is calculated by subtracting the minimal luminal diameter (MLD) value at follow-up from postprocedural MLD. LL has traditionally served as a major outcome measure in bare-metal stent (BMS) trials and continues to play a similar role in the era of DES.[4,5] However, advanced imaging techniques, such as intravascular ultrasound (IVUS)[6] and optical coherence tomography (OCT),[7,8] are increasingly the modality of choice for quantitative assessments of neointimal thickness, neointimal volume, and minimal lumen diameter MLD (see Fig. 2).

Restenosis after BMS may present itself in the form of acute coronary syndrome in up to one-third of the patients,[9,10] whereas asymptomatic patients with nonfunctional angiographic restenosis typically experience a benign course.[11] Thus, target lesion revascularization (TLR),

The authors report no disclosures or conflict of interest related to this topic.
Department of Cardiology, Harrington Heart and Vascular Institute, University Hospitals Case Medical Center, Case Western Reserve University School of Medicine, 11100 Euclid Avenue, Mailstop Lakeside 5038, Cleveland, OH 44106, USA
* Corresponding author.
E-mail address: David.Zidar@UHhospitals.org

Intervent Cardiol Clin 5 (2016) 281–293
http://dx.doi.org/10.1016/j.iccl.2016.03.002
2211-7458/16/$ – see front matter © 2016 Elsevier Inc. All rights reserved.

defined as any repeat percutaneous intervention of the treated coronary segment or bypass surgery of the target vessel, has been proposed as the most specific clinical restenosis end-point among other clinical markers (ie, death, myocardial infarction, symptoms recurrence, or combined major adverse cardiac events [MACE]).[12] Target vessel revascularization (TVR) expands the definition of TLR to include repeat percutaneous intervention of the target vessel, irrespective of the location of the stenosis within the treated segment. Target lesion failure (TLF) includes TLR, death, or myocardial infarction.

Thus, one should consider differences in time of follow-up assessment, percentage of patients with angiographic follow-up versus clinically driven data, and the patient population when interpreting clinical trial restenosis data. The incidence of LL and binary restenosis in key stent clinical trials is described in Table 1.[5,13–24]

MECHANISMS OF RESTENOSIS
Normal Versus Pathologic Response to Arterial Injury
The initial consequences of balloon angioplasty or coronary stenting are endothelial denudation, mechanical disruption of atherosclerotic plaque, often with dissection into the tunica media and occasionally adventitia, and stretch of the entire artery.[25] Endothelial injury, platelet aggregation, inflammatory cell infiltration, release of growth factors, medial smooth muscle cell (SMC) modulation and proliferation, proteoglycan deposition, and extracellular matrix (EMC) remodeling are the major milestones in the temporal sequence of the response to this trauma. In most patients, the healing response includes re-endothelialization of the artery without significant reduction in vessel diameter.

Restenosis is a pathophysiologic version of this response to injury, which leads to narrowing of the vessel segment due to negative vascular remodeling or neointimal hyperplasia (NIH)[26] (Fig. 1). NIH is initiated by multiple factors. The loss of a functional endothelium contributes NIH; endothelial injury alone is sufficient for the development of NIH in animal models,[27] through mechanisms that may require cytokine such as platelet-derived growth factor (PDGF) and transforming growth factor-β (TGF-β) to induce migration and proliferation of vascular smooth muscle cells (VSMC).[28] Platelet activation and deposition have been shown to occur almost immediately after endothelial injury in vivo[29,30] and also leads to PDGF production. Clinically, elevated platelet reactivity measured at the time of PCI has been associated with increased restenosis rates after balloon angioplasty.[31]

Endothelial Injury, Platelet Activation, Inflammation
In animal models, endothelial injury is sufficient for the development of NIH. Several mechanisms appear to directly link endothelial activation or denudation to restenosis. First, nitric oxide–mediated responses to flow and shear stress provide a protective response. Therefore, endothelial injury leads to the production of cytokines such as PDGF and TGF-β, which can induce migration and proliferation of VSMC.[28]

Endothelial response to injury also promotes platelet adhesion. Platelet activation and deposition have been shown to occur almost immediately after endothelial injury in vivo[29,30] and results in platelet production of cytokines and growth factors, including PDGF. Elevated platelet reactivity measured at the time of PCI has been associated with increased restenosis rates after balloon angioplasty.[31]

Inflammatory cell activation may also induce restenosis.[32] Innate immune responses, which have a predominance of monocyte/macrophage infiltrates, have been described. Antigen-specific adaptive immune hypersensitivity responses typified by infiltration of T cells and B cells in conjunction with eosinophils may also play a role in restenosis (reviewed in Ref.[33]).

However, the mechanisms that account for the most proximate fork in the road between a nonproliferative healing pattern and one ending in NIH are incompletely understood.

Smooth Muscle Cell Migration, Proliferation, and Extracellular Matrix Formation
Regardless of the precise initial steps, NIH ultimately results from both the inappropriate migration and the uncontrolled proliferation of VSMC (Fig. 2). VSMCs from the media and adventitia migrate into the intimal layer in response to PDGF[34] and are aided by fracture of the internal elastic membrane. Adventitial myofibroblasts also proliferate and migrate into the neointimal.[35] These cells shift from a contractile to the synthetic phenotype. In classic BMS restenosis, VSMCs proliferate from 24 hours to 2 to 3 months after vascular injury, returning to a contractile phenotype after this period. Analysis of atherectomy specimens suggests that monocyte/macrophages also proliferate within human in-stent restenotic tissue.[36]

Although cellular division is essential for the subsequent development of restenosis, so too is the synthesis of various collagen subtypes

Table 1
Summary of pivotal restenosis trial data

Study (n)	Randomized	Drug/Agent	Device Type	In-Stent LL (Time of f/u)	In-Lesion Restenosis (Time of f/u)
BMS vs PTCA					
STRESS (n = 410)	Yes	None	Palmaz-Schatz	0.74-mm (6 mo)[a]	31.6% (6 mo)
			Balloon angioplasty	0.38-mm (6 mo)[a]	42.1% (6 mo)
BENESTENT (n = 520)	Yes	None	Palmaz-Schatz	0.65-mm (6 mo)[a]	22% (6 mo)
			Balloon angioplasty	0.32-mm (6 mo)[a]	42% (6 mo)
MUSIC (n = 161)	No	None	Palmaz-Schatz	0.77-mm (6 mo)	8.3% (6 mo)
First-generation DES					
RAVEL (n = 238)	Yes	Sirolimus	BX Velocity	−0.01-mm (6 mo)	0% (6 mo)
			BX Velocity	0.8-mm (6 mo)	26.6% (6 mo)
SIRIUS (n = 1058)	Yes	Sirolimus	BX Velocity	0.17-mm (8 mo)	8.9% (9 mo)
		None	BX Velocity	1.00 mm (8 mo)	36.3% (9 mo)
TAXUS IV (n = 1314)	Yes	Paclitaxel	Express 2	0.39-mm (SR, 9 mo)	7.9% (9 mo)
		None	Express 2	0.92-mm (9 mo)	26.6% (9 mo)
REALITY (n = 1386)	Yes	Sirolimus	BX Velocity	0.09-mm (8 mo)	9.6% (8 mo)
		Paclitaxel	Express 2	0.31-mm (8 mo)	11.1% (8 mo)
SIRTAX (n = 1012)	Yes	Sirolimus	BX Velocity	0.13-mm (9 mo)	6.7% (9 mo)
		Paclitaxel	Express 2	0.25-mm (9 mo)	11.9% (9 mo)
Newer-generation DES					
ENDEAVOR II (n = 1197)	Yes	Zotarolimus	Driver	0.61-mm (9 mo)	13.2% (9 mo)
		None	Driver	1.03-mm (9 mo)	35% (9 mo)
SPIRIT III (n = 1002)	Yes 2:1	Everolimus	Vision	0.16-mm (8 mo)	2.3% (8 mo)
		Paclitaxel	Express 2	0.30-mm (8 mo)	5.7% (8 mo)
PLATINUM QCA (n = 100)	No	Everolimus	Element	0.20-mm (9 mo)	1.1% (9 mo)[b]
RESOLUTE FIM (n = 139)	No	Zotarolimus	Driver	0.22-mm (9 mo)	2.1% (9 mo)[b]
Diabetes trials					
DIABETES-I (n = 160)	Yes	Sirolimus	BX Velocity	0.08 (9 mo)	7.7% (9 mo)
		None	BX Velocity	0.66-mm (9 mo)	33% (9 mo)
DIABETES-II (n = 80)	No	Paclitaxel	Express 2	0.42-mm (9 mo)	7.6% (9 mo)
ISAR-DIABETES (n = 250)	Yes	Sirolimus	BX Velocity	0.19-mm (6 mo)	6.9% (6 mo)
	Yes	Paclitaxel	Express 2	0.49-mm (6 mo)	16.5% (6 mo)

Abbreviations: PTCA, percutaneous transluminal coronary angioplasty.
[a] These measurements reflect "In-lesion" LL instead of "In-stent".
[b] These measurements reflect "In-segment" restenosis instead of "In-lesion".
From Zidar DA, Costa MA, Simon DI. Restenosis. In: Topol E, editor. Textbook of interventional cardiology. 7th edition. Philadelphia: Elsevier; 2016; with permission.

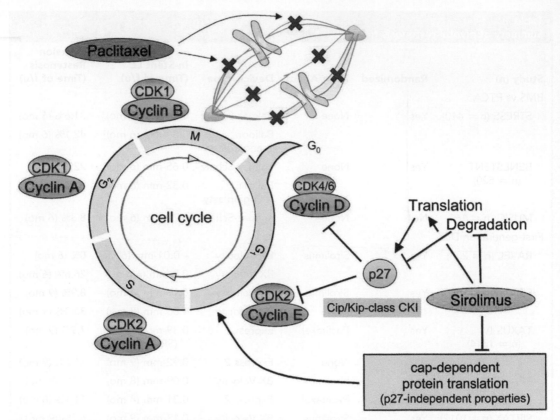

Fig. 1. Schematic representation of the VSMC cycle and regulatory mediators. The mechanism of action for pacli-taxel involves cell cycle arrest at M phase through its inhibition of microtubule assembly. Sirolimus drugs act to in-crease p27 expression with resultant arrest at G$_1$ phase. CDK, cyclin-dependent kinase; CKI, cyclin-kinase inhibitor; G1, Gap 1; G2, Gap 2; M, Mitosis; S, Synthesis. (*From* Wessley R, Schömig A, Kastrati A. Sirolimus and paclitaxel on polymer-based drug-eluting stents: similar but different. J Am Coll Cardiol 2006;47:710; with permission.)

and proteoglycans.[37] At some point, the artery enters a phase of remodeling involving ECM protein degradation and resynthesis. This final phase results in a shift in which ECM and not cellular elements become the major component of the restenotic lesion; NIH ultimately becomes tissue with relatively low cellularity.[38]

CLINICAL FEATURES OF RESTENOSIS
Predictors of Restenosis
Several procedural and clinical features have consistently predicted BMS restenosis in human studies[39–41] (Box 1). Diabetes mellitus increases the risk of restenosis whether it be after balloon an-gioplasty, BMS, or DES implantation.[42] Anatomic features, including saphenous vein graft disease, small vessel diameter, and chronic total occlusion, are associated with higher incidence of angio-graphic restenosis.[41,43–46] Although nonmodifi-able, these features are important to recognize, particularly when considering BMS versus DES.

Perhaps the most important modifiable pre-dictor of restenosis, even in the DES era, remains final luminal diameter and thus the degree of stent expansion. Angiographic and IVUS studies have consistently confirmed the importance of lumen size achieved at the end of the proce-dure.[47,48] Stent underexpansion predisposes to restenosis but also may be underappreciated without intravascular imaging, particularly in longer stented segments.[49] In the DES era, although vessel diameter remains a significant predictor of restenosis, the use of longer stents may not appreciably increase DES restenosis rates. This finding may be due to the fact that a greater luminal diameter can often be achieved with longer devices. In addition, longer DES may afford the operator the opportunity to cover from "normal to normal" tissue with a sin-gle stent even in more complex lesions.

Another technical factor that appears to in-crease restenosis rates, particularly in the DES era, is failure to cover balloon-treated segments with DES, so-called longitudinal geographic miss (LGM). LGM may occur as frequently as in 50% of cases and increases TVR greater than 2-fold.[50]

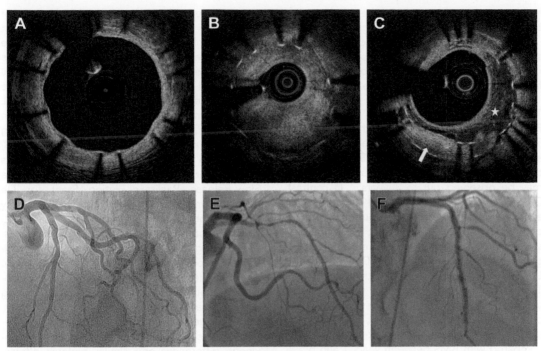

Fig. 2. Variable neointimal patterns as revealed by OCT. An OCT cross-sectional image of an everolimus-eluting stent shows complete strut coverage without evidence of ISR at 9 months follow-up (A). ISR with a typical homogeneous fibrotic neointima is typically observed after BMS and can also be observed after DES, as seen in this example, 6 years after sirolimus-eluting stent implantation (B). Atypical patterns of ISR can also been seen after DES (C). Example of a heterogeneous, low-intensity neointima within an everolimus-eluting stent (star), 1 year after implantation to treat ISR of Tacrolimus-eluting stent (arrow) implanted 4 years earlier. Corresponding angiograms for the vessel depicted by OCT are shown (D–F, respectively).

Box 1
Clinical and angiographic predictors of bare-metal stent restenosis

Diabetes mellitus

Nonsmoking status

Female gender

Acute coronary syndrome

Previous PCI

Small vessel diameter

Lesion length greater than 20 mm

Multiple stents

American College of Cardiology/American Heart Association type C lesion

Ostial location

From Zidar DA, Simon DI. Medscape education cardiology. Next-generation drug-eluting stents strut their stuff: delivering hype or hope? 2012. Available at: www.medscape.org/viewarticle/769577. Accessed January 29, 2016.

Patterns of Restenosis

In-stent restenosis (ISR) can be characterized angiographically into 1 of 4 patterns. Major distinctions revolve around whether the lesion is focal (pattern I) or diffuse (>10 mm). Diffuse ISR may be fully intrastent (pattern II), proliferative (pattern III, extending outside the stent), or resulting in total occlusion (pattern IV). Focal restenosis occurred in 42% of patients, diffuse in 21%, proliferative in 30%, and total occlusion in 7% after Palmaz-Schatz stent implantation.[51,52]

The distribution of ISR has changed with DES and may be specific to a given device. For example, restenosis after sirolimus-eluting stents (SES) is mostly (>90%) focal and usually located at the stent edges,[53,54] whereas diffuse intimal proliferation or total occlusion accounts for approximately half of the restenosis cases after polymer-coated paclitaxel-eluting stents (PES).[55]

Biological and anatomic factors may also drive particular patterns. For example, diffuse patterns of ISR are seen in more challenging clinical scenarios such as prior in-stent BMS, bypass graft disease, or diabetes mellitus. Restenosis after bifurcation PCI is frequently associated with focal stenosis at the ostium of the side branch.[56] LGM is associated with focal edge restenosis.[50]

OCT imaging, with its ability to characterize the severity, distribution, and composition of a given restenotic lesion, provides additional insight and facilitates treatment planning (see Fig. 2).

Time Course of Restenosis

BMS restenosis tends to occur within the first 6 to 9 months after implantation. Paradoxically, small angiographic studies from the BMS era suggested that after 6 months, improvements in luminal area may be observed out to 3 years.[57] In contrast, DES restenosis and its associated TLF tend follow a more linear trajectory, and thus, most events occur after 6 months. In contrast to BMS studies suggesting lumen gain after 6 months, serial angiographic studies of first-generation DES suggest that LL, albeit modest, may occur in both PES and SES.[58] The mechanisms that account for this "late catch-up" phenomena are poorly understood.[58,59] The clinical significance is also unclear, because similar rates of TLF were observed in first-generation DES compared with BMS between years 1 and 5.[60,61] Thus, the benefit of first-generation DES over BMS appears to be largely confined to the first year.

Both short- and intermediate-term TLF rates are substantially improved in the modern DES era. For instance, 5-year results from SPIRIT III (Comparison of an Everolimus-Eluting Stent and a Paclitaxel-Eluting Stent in Patients with Coronary Artery Disease) showed reductions in TLF with the Xience EES (Abbott Vascular, Santa Clara, CA, USA) compared with the Taxus PES (Boston Scientific, Natick, MA, USA) (12.7% vs 19.0%, P = .008). Similarly, the COMPARE trial (Second-generation Everolimus-eluting and Paclitaxel-eluting Stents in Real-life Practice) demonstrates improved TLF rates at 5 years with the Xience EES compared with the Taxus PES in real-world patients (11.4% vs 15.9%, P<.01).[62]

Given the lower rates and longer time course of stent failure in the DES era, it is likely that DES "restenosis" involves multiple mechanisms in addition those that drive classic BMS restenosis. For instance, the recognition that the late DES restenosis can often be accompanied by thin cap atheroma, and unstable coronary syndromes highlight the increasing overlap between classic restenosis, neoatherosclerosis, and stent thrombosis in this modern era.[63–65]

PREVENTING RESTENOSIS: STENT EVOLUTION AND DESIGN
Drug Elution
Given the unregulated nature of VSMC proliferation in the setting of NIH, several antiproliferative agents were studied in early preclinical models of restenosis. Sirolimus and paclitaxel disrupt cellular proliferation through inhibition of the G_1/S phase and M phase, respectively (see Fig. 1). These agents proved efficacious in animal models and could be delivered locally.[66–68] These 2 agents then resulted in striking reductions in LL and angiographic restenosis during first-in-human testing,[69,70] culminating in the sirolimus-eluting stent in de novo native coronary lesions (SIRIUS) and TAXUS trials (Six- and Twelve-Month Results From a Randomized, Double-Blind, Trial on a Slow-Release Paclitaxel-Eluting Stent for De Novo Lesions), confirming the impressive efficacy of the Cypher (Cordis Corporation, Miami, FL) and Taxus stents, respectively, against restenosis. These first-generation devices provided an unambiguous proof of principle that local drug delivery, to induce cell cycle arrest in the coronary endothelium, could prevent restenosis, thus ushering in a new era interventional cardiology.

Newer-generation DES use derivatives of sirolimus, engineered to have only minimal pharmacokinetic differences and similar biologic effects. Both the Endeavor and Resolute stents use zotarolimus. The chemical structure of zotarolimus differs from sirolimus at the carbon 40 position in which a tetrazole substitution is made in place of the hydroxyl group of sirolimus. This modification does not alter VSMC effects. It does, however, lead to more lipophilicity and a shorter half-life compared with sirolimus.[71] The in vivo potency of zotarolimus was 4-fold less than sirolimus when studied in assays of immunosupression in rats.[71] In a porcine model of restenosis, zotarolimus-eluting stents led to effective inhibition of NIH compared with stents containing polymer only.[71]

Everolimus is also a sirolimus analogue with a 2-hydroxyethyl substitution at position 40. It results in decreased in vitro potency but similar in vivo efficacy in immunosuppression and transplant models.[72,73] This compound was developed by Novartis and is licensed for use in both the Xience V (Abbott Vascular) and the Promus (Boston Scientific, Natick, MA, USA) DES.

For a complete discussion of anti-proliferative drug therapy for the prevention of restenosis, please also (see Habib A, Finn AV: Anti-Proliferative Drugs for Restenosis Prevention, in this issue).

Polymer and Elution Kinetics
Early clinical studies with DES showed that efficacy against restenosis was also highly dependent on the kinetics of drug delivery.[21,74] Polymers were needed to attach drug to the stent during processing, sterilization, and

storage, but also allow controlled drug delivery on stent implantation.

The polymer design used in the Cypher DES consists of 3 layers. The steel struts are coated with a primer layer of Parylene C. Sirolimus is contained in a middle layer of 67% polyethylene-co-vinyl acetate (PEVA) and 33% poly-n-butyl methacrylate (PBMA) dissolved in the organic solvent tetrahydrofuran. This system leads to controlled elution of sirolimus over 30 to 60 days.[75]

The Taxus stent had a polymer composed of polystyrene-b-isobutylene-b-styrene (SIBS; Translute). Preclinical testing of the kinetics of paclitaxel elution from SIBS show that the drug is eluted as an initial burst of drug release via dissolution within the first 48 hours, followed by slow release over 10 days through diffusion from the polymer.[76] Complete drug elution from SIBS extends out to 90 days.

The polymer used in the Endeavor (Medtronic, Minneapolis, MN, USA) stent system is designed to provide more rapid drug elution. The polymer is based on biomimicry of phosphorylcholine (PC), a phospholipid found on red blood cells, to optimize the biocompatibility of the surface coating. Four PC-based monomers are cross-linked to achieve adequate adhesion and durability.[77] Biocompatibility testing in porcine coronary arteries shows no differences in endothelialization or inflammatory changes after PC-coated stent implantation compared with uncoated stents.[78–80]

The Xience V/Promus stent is designed to capitalize on the apparent biocompatibility of fluorinated surfaces. Several reports suggest fluoropassive coatings offer improved long-term biocompatibility.[81] The stent is first coated with a primer layer consisting of PBMA. The polymer is a single phase layer of 7.8 μm consisting of an 83%/17% mixture of the semicrystalline polyvinylidene fluoride-co-hexafluoropropylene and everolimus. The elution of everolimus occurs over the course of 4 months, with 25% released within the first day and an additional 50% released over the first month.[82] In a rabbit model, the Xience V stent design resulted in improved endothelialization compared with first-generation DES.[83]

The Resolute stent (Medtronic, Minneapolis, MN) uses a novel polymer system termed Bio-Linx, which is designed to extend the drug elution of zolatrolimus compared with the Endeavor system. This formulation of 3 copolymers consists of a hydrophilic C19 polymer, polyvinyl pyrrolidone, and a hydrophobic C10 polymer, combined in a ratio of 63%/10%/27%. The stent is covered with a primer coat of Parylene C, and then zotarolimus is added in a drug/polymer ratio of 35%/65%. This formulation leads to an elution profile from the Resolute DES in which 85% of zotarolimus elutes within 60 days, and the remainder elutes by 180 days.[84] In contrast, 98% of zotarolimus elutes within 14 days from the PC-based polymer on the Endeavor DES.[85] Due in part to its hydrophilic surface, the BioLinx appears to be inert relative to other DES polymers when tested using a novel in vitro screening system.[86]

For a complete discussion of polymer and elution kinetics, please also (see Tzafriri AR, Edelman ER: Endovascular Drug Delivery and Drug Elution Systems: First Principles, in this issue).

Scaffold Redesign

BMS and first-generation DES were mounted on stainless steel platforms with relatively large strut sizes. For instance, the Cypher stent used 316L stainless steel, and a strut thickness of 140 μm. The first-generation Taxus was also manufactured with 316L stainless steel and had a strut thickness of 132 μm. Although this stainless steel had an extensive safety track record and provided excellent radial strength, the bulky design of these stainless steel stents also limited deliverability to distal, calcified, or tortuous segments. The development of cobalt chromium and platinum alloys for BMS platforms has allowed for substantial reductions in strut thickness with preserved radial strength.[87]

Early preclinical studies suggested that restenotic responses may be affected by certain biomechanical aspects (architecture, material composition, and strut thickness) of the stent, independent of vessel injury.[88,89] Several randomized trials now support the notion that stent characteristics, particularly strut size, may affect the risk of restenosis.[90,91] For instance, the ISAR-STEREO 2 (Intracoronary stenting and angiographic results: strut thickness effect on restenosis outcome) trial showed that use of the thin strut (50 μm) RX multilink (Guidant, Advanced Cardiovascular Systems, Santa Clara, CA) resulted in marked reduction in binary restenosis and TVR (12.3% vs 21.9%) compared with the thick strut (140 μm) BX velocity (Cordis Corporation, Miami, FL).[91] Next-generation DES have taken advantage of these advances in stent design (see Table 1), and this may account for improved outcomes associated with newer DES compared with their first-generation counterparts.

An important limitation of durable polymer DES is the rare but potentially catastrophic late and very late stent thrombosis. Studies investigating this pathologic entity have demonstrated hypersensitivity, delayed healing, and incomplete neointimal coverage, which many have attributed to the presence of the durable polymer.[12–14] This presence has led to the development of bioresorbable polymer DES, wherein the polymer undergoes complete degradation over time, essentially leaving behind a BMS. Although several bioresorbable polymer DES have been designed to date, the SYNERGY (Boston Scientific, Natick MA, USA), everolimus-eluting, bioresorbable polymer stent is perhaps the most applicable in the current era of DES. The EVOLVE II (Efficacy and Safety of a Novel Bioabsorbable Polymer-Coated, Everolimus-Eluting Coronary Stent) trial sought to determine the effectiveness of the SYNERGY stent by randomizing patients in 1:1 fashion to either the SYNERGY stent or the Promus Element EES.[15] The 1-year TLF rates were similar in the 2 groups, confirming noninferiority of the SYNERGY stent.

For a complete discussion of stent platforms, please also (see Partida RA, Yeh RW: Contemporary Drug Eluting Stent Platforms: Design, Safety, and Clinical Efficacy, in this issue).

TREATMENT OF RESTENOSIS
After Percutaneous Transluminal Coronary Angioplasty
Restenosis after balloon angioplasty alone should typically be treated with stenting when technically feasible, given randomized data showing improved angiographic and clinical results compared with repeat balloon angioplasty alone.[92] Stenting in this scenario may yield similarly durable results compared with stenting of de novo lesions.

After Bare-Metal Stent
Before DES, in-stent BMS restenosis was associated with high rates of repeat TLR.[93] For instance, Mehran and colleagues[51] showed that TLR rates after treatment of BMS restenosis depended on the pattern of restenosis and ranged from 19.1% for focal lesions, compared with 50% for proliferative lesions, and to 83.4% for total occlusions.

Intracoronary radiation results in improved early TVR rates (26% vs 68%), but higher rates of TLR between 6 months and 5 years (21.5% vs 6.1%).[94] Brachytherapy is also associated with very late stent thrombosis, probably becasue of delayed endothelial healing.[95] The introduction of DES has significantly improved the treatment of BMS restenosis. For instance, first-generation DES have each been shown to be superior to balloon angioplasty as well as brachytherapy for the treatment of BMS restenosis.[96–99] Observational trials of contemporary DES designs

suggest these newer devices also lead to durable results with low restenosis and MACE rates (10%–15% at 9–12 months).[100,101] Thus, optimal treatment of BMS restenosis, especially proliferative lesions, will typically involve restenting with DES. The development of drug-eluting balloon technology represents another potential technologic advance that may impact restenosis treatment in the near future.[102]

After Drug-Eluting Stent
Despite its lower frequency compared with BMS, when DES restenosis occurs, it is associated with poor long-term outcomes with recurrence rates of 18% to 51%. Similar to BMS, the rate of treatment failure for DES restenosis depends on the pattern of restenosis, with the highest repeat restenosis rates observed in patients with diffuse patterns.[103,104]

Observational studies suggest repeat DES may be preferable to balloon angioplasty alone, even for focal lesions.[105] The ISAR-DESIRE 2 (Randomized Trial of Paclitaxel- Versus Sirolimus-Eluting Stents for Treatment of Coronary Restenosis in Sirolimus-Eluting Stents) trial compared repeat stenting with SES or PES in patients with SES restenosis.[106] These first-generation DES were equally effective at treating DES restenosis; however, TLR rates ($\approx$15.5%) were relatively high in both groups. Stent thrombosis (0.4% SES vs 0.4% PES; P>.99) was similar between both stents. Intravascular brachytherapy may lead to additional improvements in TLR when added to repeat treatment with DES,[107] but is not widely used in contemporary practice given concerns for late thrombotic events. A potential role exists for drug-eluting balloons in treating DES restenosis, especially when recurrence has great theoretic appeal, but additional studies are needed.[108]

Debulking and Other Plaque-Modifying Modalities
Numerous dubulking/plaque-modifying devices have been used for lesion modification at the time of repeat intervention for ISR. Laser atherectomy relies on high-intensity light, heat, and shock waves for ablation of tissue and may facilitate greater expansion on stent delivery. Rotational atherectomy uses a diamond-tipped burr, rotating at high speeds, to mechanically debulk the lesion. The cutting balloon, with its 3 to 4 blades on the outer surface, makes cuts along the endothelium on expansion and purportedly improves dilatability of the intended segment. The angiosculpt scoring balloon has nitinol struts, which encircle the balloon to

facilitate complete expansion of ISR tissue. These devices each have been shown to result in greater luminal diameter, but this has not consistently resulted in demonstrable improvements in clinical event rates in the pre-DES era.[109–111] Additional study is needed, however, to determine the efficacy and optimal manner of debulking in the current DES era.

SUMMARY AND FUTURE DIRECTIONS

Restenosis is a pathologic response to vessel injury during PCI. Iterative improvements in stent technology, including thinner struts and drug elution, have led to impressive reductions in the rates of restenosis over the past 2 decades. Nevertheless, even in the current era, restenosis persists as the major cause of stent failure.

The future evolution of PCI technology, as it relates to restenosis, will be greatly impacted in the near future by studies of both bioresorbable technologies and drug-eluting balloons. Each has the potential to be game changers for interventional cardiology, adding additional tools for both complex and routine clinical scenarios.

Only time will tell if this next era of evolution is a panacea or another stepping stone. However, the experience over the last 4 decades should serve as a reminder. Coronary atherosclerosis is a formidable adversary, and despite exciting recent developments, the current and next generation of devices, no matter how improved, are also unlikely to be the last.

REFERENCES

1. Gruntzig AR, Senning A, Siegenthaler WE. Nonoperative dilatation of coronary-artery stenosis: percutaneous transluminal coronary angioplasty. N Engl J Med 1979;301(2):61–8.
2. Roubin GS, King SB 3rd, Douglas JS Jr. Restenosis after percutaneous transluminal coronary angioplasty: the Emory University Hospital experience. Am J Cardiol 1987;60(3):39B–43B.
3. Ruygrok PN, Webster MW, de Valk V, et al. Clinical and angiographic factors associated with asymptomatic restenosis after percutaneous coronary intervention. Circulation 2001;104(19):2289–94.
4. Mehilli J, Kastrati A, Wessely R, et al. Randomized trial of a nonpolymer-based rapamycin-eluting stent versus a polymer-based paclitaxel-eluting stent for the reduction of late lumen loss. Circulation 2006;113(2):273–9.
5. Morice MC, Serruys PW, Sousa JE, et al. A randomized comparison of a sirolimus-eluting stent with a standard stent for coronary revascularization. N Engl J Med 2002;346(23):1773–80.
6. Garcia-Garcia HM, Shen Z, Piazza N. Study of restenosis in drug eluting stents: new insights from greyscale intravascular ultrasound and virtual histology. EuroIntervention 2009;5(Suppl D):D84–92.
7. Yamamoto M, Takano M, Murakami D, et al. Optical coherence tomography analysis for restenosis of drug-eluting stents. Int J Cardiol 2011;146(1):100–3.
8. Bezerra HG, Costa MA, Guagliumi G, et al. Intracoronary optical coherence tomography: a comprehensive review clinical and research applications. JACC Cardiovasc Interv 2009;2(11):1035–46.
9. Chen MS, John JM, Chew DP, et al. Bare metal stent restenosis is not a benign clinical entity. Am Heart J 2006;151(6):1260–4.
10. Rathore S, Kinoshita Y, Terashima M, et al. A comparison of clinical presentations, angiographic patterns and outcomes of in-stent restenosis between bare metal stents and drug eluting stents. EuroIntervention 2010;5(7):841–6.
11. Popma JJ, van den Berg EK, Dehmer GJ. Long-term outcome of patients with asymptomatic restenosis after percutaneous transluminal coronary angioplasty. Am J Cardiol 1988;62(17):1298–9.
12. Kuntz RE, Baim DS. Defining coronary restenosis. Newer clinical and angiographic paradigms. Circulation 1993;88(3):1310–23.
13. Serruys PW, de Jaegere P, Kiemeneij F, et al. A comparison of balloon-expandable-stent implantation with balloon angioplasty in patients with coronary artery disease. Benestent Study Group. N Engl J Med 1994;331(8):489–95.
14. Fischman DL, Leon MB, Baim DS, et al. A randomized comparison of coronary-stent placement and balloon angioplasty in the treatment of coronary artery disease. Stent Restenosis Study Investigators. N Engl J Med 1994;331(8):496–501.
15. de Jaegere P, Mudra H, Figulla H, et al. Intravascular ultrasound-guided optimized stent deployment. Immediate and 6 months clinical and angiographic results from the Multicenter Ultrasound Stenting in Coronaries Study (MUSIC Study). Eur Heart J 1998;19(8):1214–23.
16. Moses JW, Leon MB, Popma JJ, et al. Sirolimus-eluting stents versus standard stents in patients with stenosis in a native coronary artery. N Engl J Med 2003;349(14):1315–23.
17. Stone GW, Ellis SG, Cox DA, et al. A polymer-based, paclitaxel-eluting stent in patients with coronary artery disease. N Engl J Med 2004;350(3):221–31.

18. Fajadet J, Wijns W, Laarman GJ, et al. Randomized, double-blind, multicenter study of the Endeavor zotarolimus-eluting phosphorylcholine-encapsulated stent for treatment of native coronary artery lesions: clinical and angiographic results of the ENDEAVOR II trial. Circulation 2006;114(8):798–806.

19. Sabate M, Jimenez-Quevedo P, Angiolillo DJ, et al. Randomized comparison of sirolimus-eluting stent versus standard stent for percutaneous coronary revascularization in diabetic patients: the diabetes and sirolimus-eluting stent (DIABETES) trial. Circulation 2005;112(14): 2175–83.

20. Kastrati A, Dibra A, Eberle S, et al. Sirolimus-eluting stents vs paclitaxel-eluting stents in patients with coronary artery disease: meta-analysis of randomized trials. JAMA 2005;294(7): 819–25.

21. Colombo A, Drzewiecki J, Banning A, et al. Randomized study to assess the effectiveness of slow- and moderate-release polymer-based paclitaxel-eluting stents for coronary artery lesions. Circulation 2003;108(7):788–94.

22. Windecker S, Remondino A, Eberli FR, et al. Sirolimus-eluting and paclitaxel-eluting stents for coronary revascularization. N Engl J Med 2005; 353(7):653–62.

23. Morice MC, Colombo A, Meier B, et al. Sirolimus- vs paclitaxel-eluting stents in de novo coronary artery lesions: the REALITY trial: a randomized controlled trial. JAMA 2006;295(8):895–904.

24. Stone GW, Midei M, Newman W, et al. Comparison of an everolimus-eluting stent and a paclitaxel-eluting stent in patients with coronary artery disease: a randomized trial. JAMA 2008; 299(16):1903–13.

25. Welt FG, Rogers C. Inflammation and restenosis in the stent era. Arterioscler Thromb Vasc Biol 2002;22(11):1769–76.

26. Forrester JS, Fishbein M, Helfant R, et al. A paradigm for restenosis based on cell biology: clues for the development of new preventive therapies. J Am Coll Cardiol 1991;17(3):758–69.

27. Koskinas KC, Chatzizisis YS, Antoniadis AP, et al. Role of endothelial shear stress in stent restenosis and thrombosis: pathophysiologic mechanisms and implications for clinical translation. J Am Coll Cardiol 2012;59(15):1337–49.

28. Palumbo R, Gaetano C, Antonini A, et al. Different effects of high and low shear stress on platelet-derived growth factor isoform release by endothelial cells: consequences for smooth muscle cell migration. Arterioscler Thromb Vasc Biol 2002;22(3):405–11.

29. Massberg S, Enders G, Leiderer R, et al. Platelet-endothelial cell interactions during ischemia/ reperfusion: the role of P-selectin. Blood 1998; 92(2):507–15.

30. Massberg S, Gawaz M, Grüner S, et al. A crucial role of glycoprotein VI for platelet recruitment to the injured arterial wall in vivo. J Exp Med 2003; 197(1):41–9.

31. Bach R, Jung F, Kohsiek I, et al. Factors affecting the restenosis rate after percutaneous transluminal coronary angioplasty. Thromb Res 1994; 74(Suppl 1):S55–67.

32. Libby P, Schwartz D, Brogi E, et al. A cascade model for restenosis. A special case of atherosclerosis progression. Circulation 1992;86(6 Suppl): III47–52.

33. Byrne RA, Joner M, Kastrati A. Polymer coatings and delayed arterial healing following drug-eluting stent implantation. Minerva Cardioangiol 2009;57(5):567–84.

34. Libby P, Warner SJ, Salomon RN, et al. Production of platelet-derived growth factor-like mitogen by smooth-muscle cells from human atheroma. N Engl J Med 1988;318(23):1493–8.

35. Scott NA, Cipolla GD, Ross CE, et al. Identification of a potential role for the adventitia in vascular lesion formation after balloon overstretch injury of porcine coronary arteries. Circulation 1996;93(12):2178–87.

36. Rogers C, Seifert P, Edelman ER. The neointima provoked by human coronary stenting: contributions of smooth muscle and inflammatory cells and extracellular matrix in autopsy specimens over time. Circulation 1998;98:I182.

37. Riessen R, Isner JM, Blessing E, et al. Regional differences in the distribution of the proteoglycans biglycan and decorin in the extracellular matrix of atherosclerotic and restenotic human coronary arteries. Am J Pathol 1994;144(5):962–74.

38. Schwartz RS, Huber KC, Murphy JG, et al. Restenosis and the proportional neointimal response to coronary artery injury: results in a porcine model. J Am Coll Cardiol 1992;19(2):267–74.

39. Singh M, Gersh BJ, McClelland RL, et al. Clinical and angiographic predictors of restenosis after percutaneous coronary intervention. Circulation 2004;109(22):2727–31.

40. Elezi SKA, Pache J, Wehinger A, et al. Diabetes mellitus and the clinical and angiographic outcome after coronary stent placement. J Am Coll Cardiol 1998;32(7):1866–73.

41. Kastrati A, Schömig Md A, Elezi Md S, et al. Predictive factors of restenosis after coronary stent placement. J Am Coll Cardiol 1997;30(6): 1428–36.

42. Abizaid A, Kornowski R, Mintz GS, et al. The influence of diabetes mellitus on acute and late clinical outcomes following coronary stent implantation. J Am Coll Cardiol 1998;32(3):584–9.

43. Hirshfeld JW Jr, Schwartz JS, Jugo R, et al. Restenosis after coronary angioplasty: a multivariate statistical model to relate lesion and procedure variables to restenosis. The M-HEART Investigators. J Am Coll Cardiol 1991;18(3):647–56.

44. Foley DP, Melkert R, Serruys PW. Influence of coronary vessel size on renarrowing process and late angiographic outcome after successful balloon angioplasty. Circulation 1994;90(3):1239–51.

45. Violaris AG, Melkert R, Serruys PW. Long-term luminal renarrowing after successful elective coronary angioplasty of total occlusions. A quantitative angiographic analysis. Circulation 1995;91(8): 2140–50.

46. Kastrati A, Elezi S, Dirschinger J, et al. Influence of lesion length on restenosis after coronary stent placement. Am J Cardiol 1999;83(12):1617–22.

47. de Feyter PJ, Kay P, Disco C, et al. Reference chart derived from post-stent-implantation intravascular ultrasound predictors of 6-month expected restenosis on quantitative coronary angiography. Circulation 1999;100(17):1777–83.

48. Serruys PW, Kay IP, Disco C, et al. Periprocedural quantitative coronary angiography after Palmaz-Schatz stent implantation predicts the restenosis rate at six months: results of a meta-analysis of the BElgian NEtherlands Stent study (BENESTENT) I, BENESTENT II Pilot, BENESTENT II and MUSIC trials. Multicenter Ultrasound Stent In Coronaries. J Am Coll Cardiol 1999;34(4): 1067–74.

49. Kang S-J, Mintz GS, Park D-W, et al. Mechanisms of in-stent restenosis after drug-eluting stent implantation: intravascular ultrasound analysis. Circ Cardiovasc Interv 2011;4(1):9–14.

50. Costa MA, Angiolillo DJ, Tannenbaum M, et al. Impact of stent deployment procedural factors on long-term effectiveness and safety of sirolimus-eluting stents (Final Results of the Multicenter Prospective STLLR Trial). Am J Cardiol 2008;101(12):1704–11.

51. Mehran R, Dangas G, Abizaid AS, et al. Angiographic patterns of in-stent restenosis: classification and implications for long-term outcome. Circulation 1999;100(18):1872–8.

52. Alfonso F, Cequier A, Angel J, et al. Value of the American College of Cardiology/American Heart Association angiographic classification of coronary lesion morphology in patients with in-stent restenosis. Insights from the Restenosis Intra-stent Balloon angioplasty versus elective Stenting (RIBS) randomized trial. Am Heart J 2006;151(3):681.e1–9.

53. Lemos PA, Saia F, Ligthart JM, et al. Coronary restenosis after sirolimus-eluting stent implantation: morphological description and mechanistic analysis from a consecutive series of cases. Circulation 2003;108(3):257–60.

54. Colombo A, Orlic D, Stankovic G, et al. Preliminary observations regarding angiographic pattern of restenosis after rapamycin-eluting stent implantation. Circulation 2003;107(17):2178–80.

55. Corbett SJ, Cosgrave J, Melzi G, et al. Patterns of restenosis after drug-eluting stent implantation: insights from a contemporary and comparative analysis of sirolimus- and paclitaxel-eluting stents. Eur Heart J 2006;27(19):2330–7.

56. Steigen TK, Maeng M, Wiseth R, et al. Randomized study on simple versus complex stenting of coronary artery bifurcation lesions: the Nordic bifurcation study. Circulation 2006;114(18): 1955–61.

57. Kimura T, Yokoi H, Nakagawa Y, et al. Three-year follow-up after implantation of metallic coronary artery stents. N Engl J Med 1996;334:561–6.

58. Park KW, Kim C-H, Lee H-Y, et al. Does "late catch-up" exist in drug-eluting stents: insights from a serial quantitative coronary angiography analysis of sirolimus versus paclitaxel-eluting stents. Am Heart J 2010;159(3):446–53.e3.

59. Tajiri K, Sato A, Hoshi T, et al. Mechanisms explaining the late "catch-up" phenomenon after sirolimus-eluting stent implantation. Int J Cardiol 2014;177(1):44–5.

60. Morice MC, Serruys PW, Barragan P, et al. Long-term clinical outcomes with sirolimus-eluting coronary stents: five-year results of the RAVEL trial. J Am Coll Cardiol 2007;50(14):1299–304.

61. Weisz G, Leon MB, Holmes DR Jr, et al. Five-year follow-up after sirolimus-eluting stent implantation results of the SIRIUS (Sirolimus-Eluting Stent in De-Novo Native Coronary Lesions) Trial. J Am Coll Cardiol 2009;53(17):1488–97.

62. Smits PC, Vlachojannis GJ, McFadden EP, et al. Final 5-year follow-up of a randomized controlled trial of everolimus- and paclitaxel-eluting stents for coronary revascularization in daily practice: the COMPARE Trial (A Trial of Everolimus-Eluting Stents and Paclitaxel Stents for Coronary Revascularization in Daily Practice). JACC Cardiovasc Interv 2015;8(9):1157–65.

63. Kang SJ, Mintz GS, Akasaka T, et al. Optical coherence tomographic analysis of in-stent neoatherosclerosis after drug-eluting stent implantation. Circulation 2011;123(25):2954–63.

64. Park S-J, Kang S-J, Virmani R, et al. In-stent neoatherosclerosis: a final common pathway of late stent failure. J Am Coll Cardiol 2012;59(23): 2051–7.

65. Habara M, Terashima M, Nasu K, et al. Morphological differences of tissue characteristics between early, late, and very late restenosis lesions after first generation drug-eluting stent implantation: an optical coherence tomography study. Eur Heart J Cardiovasc Imaging 2013;14(3):276–84.

66. Suzuki T, Kopia G, Hayashi S, et al. Stent-based delivery of sirolimus reduces neointimal formation in a porcine coronary model. Circulation 2001; 104(10):1188–93.

67. Herdeg COM, Baumbach A, Blattner A, et al. Local paclitaxel delivery for the prevention of restenosis: biological effects and efficacy in vivo. J Am Coll Cardiol 2000;35(7):1969–76.

68. Klugherz BD, Llanos G, Lieuallen W, et al. Twenty-eight-day efficacy and pharmacokinetics of the sirolimus-eluting stent. Coron Artery Dis 2002; 13(3):183–8.

69. Sousa JECM, Abizaid A, Abizaid AS, et al. Lack of neointimal proliferation after implantation of sirolimus-coated stents in human coronary arteries: a quantitative coronary angiography and three-dimensional intravascular ultrasound study. Circulation 2001;103(2):192–5.

70. Grube E, Silber S, Hauptmann KE, et al. TAXUS I. Circulation 2003;107(1):38–42.

71. Chen Y-W, Smith ML, Sheets M, et al. Zotarolimus, a novel sirolimus analogue with potent anti-proliferative activity on coronary smooth muscle cells and reduced potential for systemic immuno-suppression. J Cardiovasc Pharmacol 2007;49(4): 228–35.

72. Schuler W, Sedrani R, Cottens S, et al. SDZ RAD, a new rapamycin derivative: pharmacological properties in vitro and in vivo. Transplantation 1997;64(1):36–42.

73. Sedrani R, Cottens S, Kallen J, et al. Chemical modification of rapamycin: the discovery of SDZ RAD. Transplant Proc 1998;30(5):2192–4.

74. Lansky AJ, Costa RA, Mintz GS, et al. Non-polymer-based paclitaxel-coated coronary stents for the treatment of patients with de novo coronary lesions. Circulation 2004;109(16):1948–54.

75. Sousa JE, Costa MA, Abizaid AC, et al. Sustained suppression of neointimal proliferation by sirolimus-eluting stents. Circulation 2001;104(17): 2007–11.

76. Kamath KR, Barry JJ, Miller KM. The Taxus drug-eluting stent: a new paradigm in controlled drug delivery. Adv Drug Deliv Rev 2006;58(3):412–36.

77. Parker T, Davé V, Falotico R. Polymers for drug eluting stents. Curr Pharm Des 2010;16(36): 3978–88.

78. Whelan DM, van der Giessen WJ, Krabbendam SC, et al. Biocompatibility of phos-phorylcholine coated stents in normal porcine coronary arteries. Heart 2000;83(3):338–45.

79. Lewis AL, Tolhurst LA, Stratford PW. Analysis of a phosphorylcholine-based polymer coating on a coronary stent pre- and post-implantation. Biomaterials 2002;23(7):1697–706.

80. Malik NGJ, Shepherd L, Crossman DC, et al. Phosphorylcholine-coated stents in porcine coronary arteries: in vivo assessment of biocom-patibility. J Invasive Cardiol 2001;13(3):193–201.

81. Guidoin R, Marois Y, Zhang Z, et al. The benefits of fluoropassivation of polyester arterial prostheses as observed in a canine model. ASAIO J 1994;40(3):M870–9.

82. Sheiban IVG, Bollati M, Sillano D, et al. Next-generation drug-eluting stents in coronary artery disease: focus on everolimus-eluting stent (Xience V). Vasc Health Risk Manag 2008;4(1):31–8.

83. Joner M, Nakazawa G, Finn AV, et al. Endothelial cell recovery between comparator polymer-based drug-eluting stents. J Am Coll Cardiol 2008;52(5): 333–42.

84. Meredith IT, Worthley S, Whitbourn R, et al. The next-generation endeavor resolute stent: 4-month clinical and angiographic results from the endeavor resolute first-in-man trial. EuroIntervention 2007;3(1):50–3.

85. Pinto Slottow TL, Waksman R. Overview of the 2007 Food and Drug Administration circulatory system devices panel meeting on the endeavor zotarolimus-eluting coronary stent. Circulation 2008;117(12):1603–8.

86. Hezi-Yamit A, Sullivan C, Wong J, et al. Novel high throughput polymer biocompatibility screening designed for SAR (Structure-Activity Relationship): application for evaluating polymer coatings for cardiovascular drug-eluting stents. Comb Chem High Throughput Screen 2009;12(7):664–76.

87. Stone GW, Teirstein PS, Meredith IT, et al. A prospective, randomized evaluation of a novel everolimus-eluting coronary stent: the PLATINUM (A Prospective, Randomized, Multicenter Trial to Assess an Everolimus-Eluting Coronary Stent System [PROMUS Element] for the Treatment of up to Two De Novo Coronary Artery Lesions) trial. J Am Coll Cardiol 2011;57(16):1700–8.

88. Garasic JM, Edelman ER, Squire JC, et al. Stent and artery geometry determine intimal thickening independent of arterial injury. Circulation 2000; 101(7):812–8.

89. Rogers C, Edelman ER. Endovascular stent design dictates experimental restenosis and thrombosis. Circulation 1995;91(12):2995–3001.

90. Hoffmann R, Mintz GS, Haager PK, et al. Relation of stent design and stent surface material to subsequent in-stent intimal hyperplasia in coronary arteries determined by intravascular ultrasound. Am J Cardiol 2002;89(12):1360–4.

91. Pache J, Kastrati A, Mehilli J, et al. Intracoronary stenting and angiographic results: strut thickness effect on restenosis outcome (ISAR-STEREO-2) trial. J Am Coll Cardiol 2003;41(8):1283–8.

92. Erbel R, Haude M, Hopp HW, et al. Coronary-artery stenting compared with balloon angioplasty for restenosis after initial balloon angioplasty.

Restenosis Stent Study Group. N Engl J Med 1998; 339(23):1672–8.

93. Alfonso F, Zueco J, Cequier A, et al. A randomized comparison of repeat stenting with balloon angioplasty in patients with in-stent restenosis. J Am Coll Cardiol 2003;42(5):796–805.

94. Waksman R, Ajani AE, White RL, et al. Five-year follow-up after intracoronary gamma radiation therapy for in-stent restenosis. Circulation 2004; 109(3):340–4.

95. Costa MA, Sabaté M, van der Giessen WJ, et al. Late coronary occlusion after intracoronary brachytherapy. Circulation 1999;100(8):789–92.

96. Holmes DR Jr, Teirstein P, Satler L, et al. Sirolimus-eluting stents vs vascular brachytherapy for in-stent restenosis within bare-metal stents: the SISR randomized trial. JAMA 2006;295(11): 1264–73.

97. Stone GW, Ellis SG, O'Shaughnessy CD, et al. Paclitaxel-eluting stents vs vascular brachytherapy for in-stent restenosis within bare-metal stents: the TAXUS V ISR randomized trial. JAMA 2006; 295(11):1253–63.

98. Oliver LN, Buttner PG, Hobson H, et al. A meta-analysis of randomised controlled trials assessing drug-eluting stents and vascular brachytherapy in the treatment of coronary artery in-stent restenosis. Int J Cardiol 2008;126(2):216–23.

99. Kastrati A, Mehilli J, von Beckerath N, et al. Sirolimus-eluting stent or paclitaxel-eluting stent vs balloon angioplasty for prevention of recurrences in patients with coronary in-stent restenosis: a randomized controlled trial. JAMA 2005;293(2): 165–71.

100. Carrié D, Delarche N, Piot C, et al. Everolimus-eluting stent for the treatment of bare metal in-stent restenosis: clinical and angiographic outcomes at nine-month follow-up of XERES (Xience Evaluation in bare metal stent REStenosis) trial. EuroIntervention 2014;10(6):700–8.

101. Ota H, Mahmoudi M, Torguson R, et al. Safety and efficacy of everolimus-eluting stents for bare-metal in-stent restenosis. Cardiovasc Revasc Med 2015;16(3):151–5.

102. Indermuehle A, Bahl R, Lansky AJ, et al. Drug-eluting balloon angioplasty for in-stent restenosis: a systematic review and meta-analysis of randomised controlled trials. Heart 2013;99(5):327–33.

103. Lemos PA, van Mieghem CA, Arampatzis CA, et al. Post-sirolimus-eluting stent restenosis treated with repeat percutaneous intervention: late angiographic and clinical outcomes. Circulation 2004;109(21):2500–2.

104. Cosgrave J, Melzi G, Biondi-Zoccai GG, et al. Drug-eluting stent restenosis the pattern predicts the outcome. J Am Coll Cardiol 2006;47(12): 2399–404.

105. Latib A, Mussardo M, Ielasi A, et al. Long-term outcomes after the percutaneous treatment of drug-eluting stent restenosis. JACC Cardiovasc Interv 2011;4(2):155–64.

106. Mehilli J, Byrne RA, Tiroch K, et al. Randomized trial of paclitaxel- versus sirolimus-eluting stents for treatment of coronary restenosis in sirolimus-eluting stents: the ISAR-DESIRE 2 (Intracoronary Stenting and Angiographic Results: Drug Eluting Stents for In-Stent Restenosis 2) study. J Am Coll Cardiol 2010;55(24):2710–6.

107. Torguson R, Sabate M, Deible R, et al. Intravascular brachytherapy versus drug-eluting stents for the treatment of patients with drug-eluting stent restenosis. Am J Cardiol 2006;98(10): 1340–4.

108. Agostoni P, Belkacemi A, Voskuil M, et al. Serial morphological and functional assessment of drug-eluting balloon for in-stent restenotic lesions: mechanisms of action evaluated with angiography, optical coherence tomography, and fractional flow reserve. JACC Cardiovasc Interv 2013;6(6):569–76.

109. Mehran R, Mintz GS, Satler LF, et al. Treatment of in-stent restenosis with excimer laser coronary angioplasty: mechanisms and results compared with PTCA alone. Circulation 1997;96(7):2183–9.

110. vom Dahl J, Dietz U, Haager PK, et al. Rotational atherectomy does not reduce recurrent in-stent restenosis: results of the angioplasty versus rotational atherectomy for treatment of diffuse in-stent restenosis trial (ARTIST). Circulation 2002;105(5):583–8.

111. Albiero R, Silber S, Di Mario C, et al. Cutting balloon versus conventional balloon angioplasty for the treatment of in-stent restenosis: results of the restenosis cutting balloon evaluation trial (RESCUT). J Am Coll Cardiol 2004; 43(6):943–9.

The Systems Biocompatibility of Coronary Stenting

Kumaran Kolandaivelu, MD, PhD[a,b,*], Farhad Rikhtegar, PhD[a]

KEYWORDS

- Stent biocompatibility • Bare metal stent • Drug-eluting stent • Durable polymer
- Bioresorbable polymer • Stent thrombosis • Restenosis

KEY POINTS

- Cardiovascular innovation, and the coronary stent in particular, has played a key role in advancing our understanding of biocompatibility.
- Stent biocompatibility is contextual and must be measured relative to clinical performance; what is biocompatible in some settings need not be in others.
- Along with biomaterial innovation, advances in device design, drug use, and deployment practices have made contemporary stenting a highly optimized practice.
- The trend toward lower profile and/or fully bioresorbable devices has created both challenges and opportunities to further improve clinical performance.

INTRODUCTION

The coronary stent has propelled our understanding of the term "biocompatibility" (Fig. 1A). Stents are expanded at sites of arterial blockage and mechanically reestablish blood flow. This simplicity belies the complex reactions that occur when a stent contacts living substrates, the confluence of which dictate clinical efficacy and safety. Biocompatible materials no longer seek to eliminate biological reactions, but rather to elicit the appropriate response; stents, as with all implanted devices, should perform rather than merely exist. Because ultimate performance is assessed in the patient, stent biocompatibility is the multiscale examination not only of material and cell, but of material, structure, and device in the context of cell, tissue, and organism.[1,2]

After the first placement of coronary stents in 1986,[3] stent thrombosis (ST; Fig. 1B) and in-stent restenosis (ISR; Fig. 1C) were recognized as major adverse responses.[4–7] ISR occurs in the months to years after stent placement and arises from excessive vascular smooth muscle cell (SMC) proliferation and neointimal hyperplasia.[4] Because overgrowth drives need for revascularization, ISR is a key measure of efficacy. ST, driven by local activation/accumulation of platelets and coagulant proteins, is considered the main safety index and carries risk for unheralded occlusion.[8] These processes overlap. Thrombotic mediators and recruitment of blood-borne components such as monocytes and eosinophils drive local inflammation and the SMC response.[9] Also, clotting occurs in this injured/inflamed microenvironment, of which the stent plays an

Disclosure: The authors have nothing to disclose.

Funding: This study was supported in part by grants from AHA (12FTF12080241) and unrestricted research sponsorship from Stentys, Inc. to K. Kolandaivelu, as well as from SNSF (P2EZP3_155599) and NIH (R01 GM 49039; Prof. Elazer Reuven Edelman) to F. Rikhtegar.

[a] Institute for Medical Engineering and Science, Massachusetts Institute of Technology, 77 Massachusetts Avenue, Cambridge, MA 02139, USA; [b] Cardiovascular Division, Brigham and Women's Hospital, Harvard Medical School, 75 Francis Street, Boston, MA 02115, USA

* Corresponding author. IMES Clinical Research Center, Massachusetts Institute of Technology, E25-201, 77 Massachusetts Avenue, Cambridge, MA 02139.

E-mail address: kkolandaivelu@partners.org

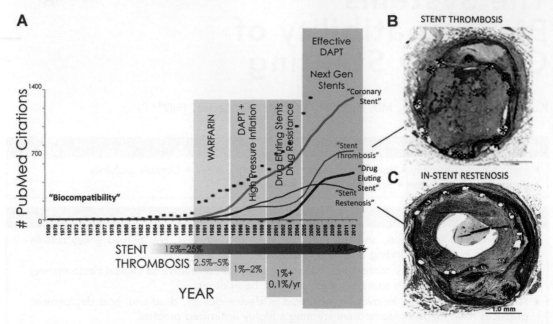

Fig. 1. (A) Annual PubMed citations for "biocompatibility" (dotted-line), and "Coronary Stent" (gray) showing their temporal association, as well as "stent thrombosis" (red) and "stent restenosis" (dark red), which emerged shortly after. Rates of stent thrombosis have been driven down from greater than 15% to less than 1%, as a result of many factors. Examples of vascular obstruction from (B) stent thrombosis and (C) in-stent restenosis as key safety and efficacy measures, respectively. DAPT, dual antiplatelet therapy. (Adapted from Alfonso F, Byrne RA, Rivero F, et al. Current treatment of in-stent restenosis. J Am Coll Cardiol 2014;63:2659–73; and Nakano M, Yahagi K, Otsuka F, et al. Causes of early stent thrombosis in patients presenting with acute coronary syndrome: an ex vivo human autopsy study. J Am Coll Cardiol 2014;63:2510–20; with permission.)

inciting but partial role.[10,11] Subendothelial components such as tissue factor and matrix ligands impinge directly on clotting pathways.[12] This complex environment varies dynamically as the body reacts, responds, and heals with reestablishment of an intact endothelial layer.

The grail of stent biocompatibility has been to find materials that resist thrombotic and inflammatory reactions while maximizing endothelialization and simultaneously providing radial support, flexibility, and radiopacity. Because many goals run counter to one another (ie, reduction of platelet adhesion at the expense of endothelial adhesion; increased radial support at the expense of higher profile, less flexible devices), biomaterial design is necessarily a process of optimization. This review tracks the major biomaterial advances in coronary stents design, and discuss biocompatibility in the context of multiparameter, optimized clinical performance.

BARE METALS AND PASSIVE MATERIALS

To meet the challenges of percutaneous deployment, metals with high moduli of elasticity and yield strengths have been a staple. Of the metals, surgical grade 316L stainless steel (SS),

recognized for its high resistance to corrosion, has served as the historical benchmark. In 2005, Sprague and Palmaz[13] reported a composite stent biocompatibility index and ranked a range of stable materials based on in vitro thromboinflammatory and endothelial cell responses. In this head-to-head comparison, SS ranked most biocompatible. Although such in vitro surrogates have debatable relevance to in vivo contexts, they carry an important implication. Despite being labeled 'biocompatible,' SS alone falls short of meeting clinical demands. Initial ST rates on SS platforms are as high as 15% to 25%.[3,5] Although this early incidence was overcome by accompanying antithrombotic strategies and improvements to stent design and interventional practices (see Fig. 1A),[5,14] ISR with SS devices persisted at rates of 20% to 30%, driving the need for biomaterial advance.[15,16]

Passive Coatings

Coatings applied to metal structures are able to impart them with beneficial surfaces while maintaining bulk properties. Overtime, even resistant metals such as 316L SS corrode and release ions (ie, nickel, chromium, and molybdenum).[17] Despite well-recognized nickel allergies, common endovascular metals such as 316L SS, cobalt chromium, or nitinol, contain significant levels of nickel (12%, 10%–35%, and 50%, respectively).[17] Fortunately, presence need not correlate with adverse response. A number of approaches can reduce the surface density of unwanted ions and prevent their release, including surface polishing, coatings such as diamondlike carbon, pyrolytic carbon, or silica carbide, or passivation with an oxide layer.[17–21] Perhaps the most clinically notable example has been the addition of a titanium–nitride–oxide layer. In addition to blocking ions, there is unsubstantiated suggestion that the nitrogenous layer may play an active role in promoting vascular health. Initial preclinical[22] and clinical data[23] demonstrated the ability for these platforms to significantly reduce ISR relative to other bare metal platforms (approximately 15% vs 30%), a finding that has allowed them to compete with more contemporary strategies of drug elution (described elsewhere in this article).[24]

A material surface does far more than gate ion release. Properties such as interfacial energy and surface topography influence biology directly,[1,18,25] yet despite decades of exploration, much remains to be understood. Upon contact with biological environments, surfaces are altered through absorption of proteins that bind in different proportions and conformations.[26,27] It is this dynamic layer, rather than the bare material per se, that impacts the evolution of biological response. Although a priori application of human plasma proteins, fibronectin, or heparin have been used to steer biological response and have been shown to provide hemocompatibilty benefits, such approaches have yet to demonstrate improved ISR.[18,21,25,28] Recently, CD34-antibody–coated surfaces have been used as another means to control the material/biological interface. By capturing circulating endothelial progenitor cells, stents incorporating these surfaces can, in theory, accelerate healing and have demonstrated noninferiority to comparator devices in first-in-man studies.[29]

Surface energy dictates device hydrophilicity and hydrophobicity, and is central when considering how proteins and cells interact with a material.[25] A variety of processes and coatings have been developed and can modify surface wettability. Efforts have led down "tri"-vergent paths from the extremes of hydrophilicity and hydrophobicity to levels in between. Favorable properties of hydrophobic coatings, as exemplified by Teflon-like fluoropolymers, are their ability to improve hemocompatibilty through reduced fibrinogen adsorption and platelet adhesion, albeit at potential expense of endothelial cell attachment (Fig. 2A).[13,30] Given the desire to integrate rather than eliminate responses, a different approach has been to create biomimetic surfaces yielding hydrophilic, phosphoryl choline (PC)-coated platforms.[30–32] PC is the major zwitterion in membrane phospholipids, and is thought to impart favorable protein and cell interactions.[26,33] Though PC surfaces are labeled "hydrophilic," their water contact angle (CA) is approximately 85° and they are best considered amphiphilic.[30] Realization of truly hydrophilic polymers has been limited traditionally by aqueous swelling and poor durability. Indeed, even amphiphilic PC-coated stent surfaces have the tendency to crack and embolize as compared with hydrophobic coatings.[30,34,35] Although in vitro evidence demonstrated reduced monocyte adhesion to these wettable polymers and early clinical studies reported promise, others maintained concerns of persistent ISR.[17,31]

More recently, ultrahydrophilic surfaces have been explored. As a case in point, when the CA varied from 56.6° to 14° through application of hydrophilic Pluronic copolymers to a polysulfone surface, albumin binding increased, fibrinogen decreased, and platelet adhesion dropped by 2 to 3 orders of magnitude.[36] Recently, a novel surface treatment applied directly to metals (Qvanteq AG) demonstrated the ability to reduce CA to less than 10°, reducing thrombogenicity and inflammation while promoting rapid endothelialization both in vitro and in vivo as compared with contemporary devices (Fig. 2B).[27,37] A clinical trial is underway to consider how these bare metal data translate into patients (clinicaltrials.gov ID: NCT02176265).

Microscale and Macroscale Features

Surface topography and roughness have also been explored as means to shape biological responses.[18,25] Smooth metal surfaces, as created through laser, chemical, magnetic, or electrolytic polishing, can provide corrosion resistance and have been widely used to reduce thrombogenicity and neointimal hyperplasia.[25] Yet, despite the seemingly intuitive benefits of a smooth surface, many examples counter this premise. Recently, laser etching 316L SS stents was shown to dramatically reduce water CA from 75° to approximately 0° and increase endothelial proliferation by 8-fold.[38] Conversely, nanotextures have led to superhydrophobic surfaces (CA >150°), the biocompatible implications of which are beginning to be explored.[39] Many other investigations have examined controlled microscale and nanoscale surface topology (pits, posts, gratings, islands, etc; Fig. 3A).[18,40,41]

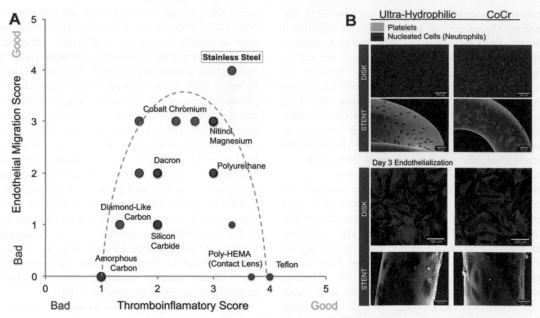

Fig. 2. (A) Side-by-side comparison of an in vitro stent biocompatibility score for durable biomaterials as judged by thromboinflammation and endothelial migration; stainless steel ranked highest. (B) Simple surface modifications to metal surfaces continue to be explored as a means of improving performance. Shown is a marked reduction in platelet adhesion, enhanced neutrophil attachment, and stable endothelial cell growth with stents undergoing ultrahydophilic treatment as compared with bare metal surfaces. CoCr, cobalt chromium; HEMA, hydroxyethyl methacrylate. (Data from Sprague EA, Palmaz JC. A model system to assess key vascular responses to biomaterials. J Endovasc Ther 2005;12:594–604.)

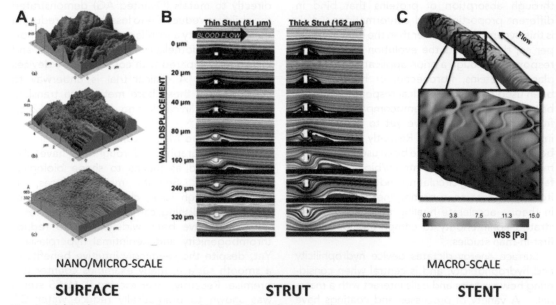

Fig. 3. Multiscale geometry plays a critical role in defining the local environment in which biocompatibility is assessed. Thus, features from the (A) nanoscale/microscale surface topology[41] to (B) strut dimensions[43] to the (C) in situ stent geometry,[49] must all be considered as components of the integrated response. (Adapted from (A) Ranjan A, Webster TJ. Increased endothelial cell adhesion and elongation on micron-patterned nano-rough poly(dimethylsiloxane) films. Nanotechnology 2009;20:305102; with permission; (B) Kolandaivelu K, Swaminathan R, Gibson WJ, et al. Stent thrombogenicity early in high-risk interventional settings is driven by stent design and deployment and protected by polymer-drug coatings. Circulation 2011;123:1400–9; with permission; (C) O'Brien CC, Kolandaivelu K, Brown J, et al. Constraining OCT with knowledge of device design enables high accuracy hemodynamic assessment of endovascular implants. PLoS One 2016;11(2):e0149178.)

Recalling the biomimicry of PC coatings, such patterning is thought to mimic the natural topology of biological tissue, promoting favorable interactions such as endothelial cell alignment, migration, and health.[18] Yet, when taken together, the diversity of studies indicate how much remains to be understood in terms of defining optimal topology. On the one hand, nanometer-scale alterations tune cellular responses, whereas on the other, even coarse sand-blasting of SS stents can yield in vivo benefits as compared with smooth surfaces.[42]

In addition to this microscale surface environment (nanometers to micrometers), the macroscale hemodynamic environment (micrometer to millimeter) established upon stent placement is impacted by a stent's bulk material properties via influence on strut geometry, stent design, and the stent's ability to serve as a vascular scaffold.[5,43–45] Because biological responses occur in this local physiologic context, the bulk material is of critical importance in defining stent biocompatibility in vivo. Indeed, among the most clinically impactful material modification to bare metal stents to date has been the use of stronger metals such as cobalt chromium and platinum chromium alloys (yield strengths of approximately 500 MPa relative to that of 316LSS of approximately 350 MPa),[17,25] which enable thinner struts (approximately 80 vs approximately 140 μm).[43] In addition to reducing foreign material presence, thinner devices are less disruptive to near-wall flow patterns (Fig. 3B, C) and can promote endothelial recovery, improving rates of ST and ISR, particularly when placed in complex lesions where risks of suboptimal deployment are greatest.[43,45–49] Robust performance gains and improved deliverability have made these chromium alloys the metals of choice. It is worth mentioning that in the biocompatibility index discussed (see Fig. 2A), cobalt chromium ranked worse than SS.[13] Acknowledging the limitations of overinterpretation, this stresses the many factors contributing to clinical biocompatibility beyond surface interaction alone (ie, strut thickness).

ACTIVE DRUG-ELUTING SURFACES

Drug-eluting stents (DES) received approval from the US Food and Drug Administration in 2003 and rapidly became the dominant means of quelling ISR.[50] Just as systemic administration of antithrombotic drugs permitted clinically acceptable rates of stent hemocompatibilty, antiproliferative drugs (in particular, sirolimus and –limus derivatives and paclitaxel), have

been central to achieving acceptable rates of ISR (<5%–15%).[4] The high toxicities associated with these chemotherapy-derived agents require use of advanced surfaces that can serve as drug reservoirs and control local release.[51]

Durable Coatings
Because drug hydrophobicity promotes tissue retention,[52,53] the durable hydrophobic polymers styrene isoprene butadiene (Taxus) and poly ethylene-co-vinyl acetate/poly butyl methacrylate (PEVA/PBMA; Cypher),[54] became favored over aqueous swelling polymers (ie, polyacrylate; QuaDS-QP2)[35] and dominated first-generation DES as a means of sustaining drug release (Fig. 4A).[55] Despite initial success in limiting ISR, concerns of prolonged ST risk surfaced in 2004 with convincing evidence by 2006.[8,56,57] Complex factors underlie this adverse signal. Prolonged tissue retention of antiproliferative drugs delay reendothelialization leading to chronic subendothelial exposure.[10,11] Moreover, the drugs augment local thrombogenicity through a variety of mechanisms, such as SMC tissue factor expression.[8] In the case of polymers such as PEVA/PBMA and polyacrylate, inflammatory responses peaked after drug elution, suggesting that the polymers themselves could induce inflammation and hypersensitivity.[35,56] Issues of antiplatelet drug nonresponsiveness also underscored the need for effective, prolonged durations of dual antiplatelet therapy, without which ST risk increased by nearly 2 orders of magnitude.[10,58] Although first-generation polymer stents were not innately thrombogenic (Fig. 4B),[43] they were in the context of delayed healing, suboptimal adjunctive treatment, and long-term biological response.

Next-generation devices were introduced to overcome the shortcomings of first-generation DES. As with their bare metal counterparts, use of stronger metals (ie, cobalt chromium, platinum chromium, composites) enable thin backbones (see Fig. 4A).[17,18,43,55] Major polymeric advances include hydrophobic strategies using polyvinylidene fluoride-hexafluoropropylene (PVDF-HFP; CA 129°) to controllably elute everolimus (Xience; Promus) as well as biomimicking PC and BioLinx polymers (CA of 81° and 94° for Endeavor and Endeavor Resolute, respectively) to elute zotarolimus.[30,54] Although PC coatings rapidly release hydrophobic drug over approximately 1 month, BioLinx was formulated to sustain release over 6 months using a blend of hydrophilic (C10 Polymer and polyvinyl pyrrolidinone) and hydrophobic (C19 Polymer) polymers.[54] Comparing these fast and slow

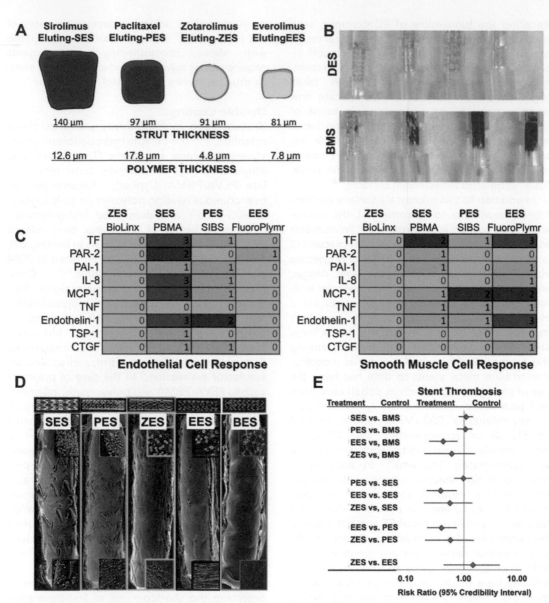

Fig. 4. (A) First-generation (SES, PES) and second-generation (ZES, EES) drug-eluting stents (DES) demonstrating reduction in thickness enabled by cobalt chromium alloys. (B) Despite concerns for stent thrombosis in first-generation devices, the platforms themselves were not thrombogenic.[43] (C) Endothelial and smooth muscle cell gene expression of prothrombotic and proinflammatory markers in response to durable polymers (green favorable, red poor; data collated from reference[54]). (D) In vivo endothelialization in a rabbit iliac model demonstrating delayed healing in first-generation SES and PES.[60] (E) Metaanalysis of randomized, controlled trials demonstrating improvements in stent thrombosis with second-generation platforms compared with bare metal and first-generation devices.[62] BMS, bare metal stent. (Adapted from (B) Kolandaivelu K, Swaminathan R, Gibson WJ, et al. Stent thrombogenicity early in high-risk interventional settings is driven by stent design and deployment and protected by polymer-drug coatings. Circulation 2011;123:1400–9; with permission; (D) Joner M, Nakazawa G, Finn AV, et al. Endothelial cell recovery between comparator polymer-based drug-eluting stents. J Am Coll Cardiol 2008;52:333–42; (E) Abizaid A, Costa JR Jr. New drug-eluting stents: an overview on biodegradable and polymer-free next generation stent systems. Circ Cardiovasc Interv 2010;3:384–93.)

zotarolimus–eluting platforms directly, the rate of 6-month uncovered struts with subconfluent endothelialization increased from 0% to 7.4% (P<.001), respectively, whereas percent obstruction decreased from 36.9% to 12.5% (P<.01).[59] These data highlight the trade-off between rapid endothelialization and ISR in optimizing drug delivery.

High-throughput biocompatibility profiling of various DES polymers in vitro supports the theoretic benefits of biomimicry in terms of reduced prothrombotic and proinflammatory endothelial cell and SMC markers (Fig. 4C). However, when tested in vivo and clinically, sustained-release next-generation DES, as a class, outperformed their first-generation predecessors with respect to healing, ISR, need for revascularization, and ST (Fig. 4D, E).[60] Moreover, accumulated clinical evidence suggests that the favorable hemocompatibilty of hydrophobic designs may even lead to a reduction in ST as compared with bare metal stents, suggesting them as a new benchmark for both stent efficacy (ISR) and safety (ST; see Fig. 4E).[61,62]

Polymer-Free and Bioresorbable Coatings

Parallel to the development of next-generation durable polymer DES, many strategies to minimize polymer presence have emerged, driven by concerns for prolonged inflammatory response to retained polymers and a potential for late ISR.[53,56] One approach is to restrict polymers to specific aspects of metallic struts such as wall contacting abluminal surfaces or macroscopic wells.[63] Alternatively, entirely polymer-free delivery methods have been explored, which leverage inorganic coatings such as hydroxyapatite (VestaSync)[64] or pyrolytic carbon (Carbofilm; OPTIMA), or microporous/nanoporous patterning of metallic surfaces from which drug elutes (YUKON).[63,65] Although some methods show potential, development is challenged by difficulties of processing, sustaining drug release, coating stability, and most important the need to show cost-effective advantages over other next-generation platforms.[66]

The most mature strategy to limit polymer presence is with use of biodegradable polymers that either fully or partially coat a metallic backbone.[66,67] The most commonly used are polylactic acid (strong, stiff, slow degradation), poly-glycolic acid (strong, very fast degradation), and their copolymer, poly-lactic-co-glycolic acid (strong, stiff, fast degradation), as well as polycaprolactone (high flexibility, medium degradation).[68] To degrade, the polymers absorb water and are then hydrolyzed and fragmented into oligomeric forms, thereby losing structural strength. These oligomers diffuse from the matrix, where they are phagocytosed and metabolized by the Krebs cycle.[69,70] Because polymer degradation occurs on a time scale of approximately year, controlled drug release can be sustained over months. However, because polymer degradation can create acidic byproducts and promote inflammation, there is a theoretic risk to their use.[71,72] Moreover, the optimal balance between drug elution and polymer degradation is not well-defined. Recent evidence shows that release of sirolimus over days in a rapidly degrading omega-3 fatty acid coating remained efficacious, attributable to sustained receptor binding and drug–tissue retention.[53] Yet, given the observed clinical trade-off in rapid endothelialization versus ISR between fast- and slow-eluting zotarolimus platforms,[59] this notion, as with all advances, must be vetted clinically. Indeed, although early evidence suggested benefits of bioresorbable coatings versus first-generation devices,[73] this no longer seems to hold when compared with contemporary durable platforms (Fig. 5A). In a metaanalysis of 106,427 patients drawn from 126 randomized trials, biodegradable coatings, although superior to bare metal stents and first-generation DES, were comparable to next-generation durable polymer devices (Fig. 5B).[66] In fact, there remained a signal for reduction in ST with durable hydrophobic-coated platforms, supported convincingly in a recent arteriovenous porcine shunt model (see Fig. 5A).[74]

SYSTEMS BIOCOMPATIBILITY AND FULL BIORESORBTION IN THE TREND OF LOW-PROFILE DEVICES

By any measure, stent biocompatibility has improved from first reporting in the *New England Journal of Medicine* when 3 clotting events occurred within weeks after placement of 24 devices,[3] to present day when it remains difficult to differentiate contemporary designs despite hundreds of thousands of patients followed over years.[66] Interwoven advances in material, design, drug, and deployment together contribute to this present-day performance. Although game-changing advance is challenged by the inherent nature of multiparameter design optimization, bioresorbable vascular scaffolds (BVS) are poised to change the game. BVS serve transiently as scaffolds, then resorb completely in the months to years after placement. As such, they raise the intriguing possibility to restore vasoactivity, provide late luminal gain, enable subsequent interventions, and even transform atherosclerotic vessels (ie, the "golden tube") rather than merely treat them.[75]

Although a fully degrading platform aligns with the contemporary "low-profile" philosophy of nonintrusive, thin devices, most BVS are substantially thicker than durable stents given the lower yield strength of available bioresorbable

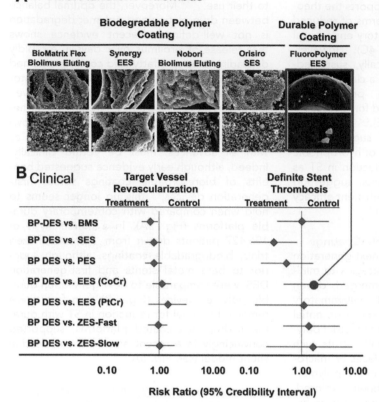

A In Vitro: Adherent Thrombus

Biodegradable Polymer Coating | Durable Polymer Coating

BioMatrix Flex Biolimus Eluting | Synergy EES | Nobori Biolimus Eluting | Orisiro SES | FluoroPolymer EES

B Clinical

Target Vessel Revascularization — Treatment / Control

Definite Stent Thrombosis — Treatment / Control

- BP-DES vs. BMS
- BP DES vs. SES
- BP DES vs. PES
- BP DES vs. EES (CoCr)
- BP DES vs. EES (PtCr)
- BP DES vs. ZES-Fast
- BP DES vs. ZES-Slow

0.10   1.00   10.00   0.10   1.00   10.00

Risk Ratio (95% Credibility Interval)

Fig. 5. (A) Porcine arteriovenous shunt model demonstrating significantly less thrombosis on a durable fluoropolymer as compared with 4 biodegradable drug-eluting stent (BD-DES) coatings.[74] (B) Metaanalysis of 126 randomized controlled trials showing BP-DES offer clinical improvements over first-generation DES and bare metal stents (BMS), although not compared with next-generation durable DES.[66] CoCr, cobalt chromium. (Adapted from Kolandaivelu K, Swaminathan R, Gibson WJ, et al. Stent thrombogenicity early in high-risk interventional settings is driven by stent design and deployment and protected by polymer-drug coatings. Circulation 2011;123:1400–9; and Bangalore S, Toklu B, Amoroso N, et al. Bare metal stents, durable polymer drug eluting stents, and biodegradable polymer drug eluting stents for coronary artery disease: mixed treatment comparison metaanalysis. BMJ 2013;347:f6625; with permission.)

materials (Fig. 6A). Many rely on the polylactic acid and poly-lactic-co-glycolic acid polymers used in bioresorbable coatings. However, in the absence of a metallic backbone, these polymers have tensile strengths of approximately 50 MPa and are prone to suboptimal radial support and variable deployment, despite the use of structures with high strut surface area/vessel surface area ratio (Fig. 6B).[76,77] Biocorrodible metals such as magnesium and iron may offer an intermediate solution, although current formulations also remain weaker than stable chromium alloys and continue to require thicker strut designs. Moreover, degradable metals reintroduce issues related to the biological impact of metal corrosion that must also be overcome.[78] Despite the allure of BVS, whose major value propositions will take years to manifest, initial clinical data suggest that first-generation devices are again associated with higher rates of early ST compared with contemporary DES (Fig. 6C).[79]

As we consider the trajectory taken by coronary stents to achieve biocompatibility (see Fig. 1A), it is important to resist the notion

that coronary scaffolds (even first generation) are inherently bioincompatible. Stents required not only generations of devices, but also coevolution of practice to achieve the excellent outcomes observable today. Although early scaffold performance might indeed be suboptimal compared with that of contemporary stents, this is in the context of the confluence of parameters that have been optimized for stents. From a systems perspective, if an optimized device changes, it is rational that the network surrounding the device (ie, drug, deployment criteria, etc) must also readapt to regain optimal "biocompatibility." As history repeats itself, there is little doubt that future use of BVS will yield improved performance as devices are rendered clinically biocompatible through a confluence of biomaterial advance, structural design, optimized drug regimens, and detailed understanding of long-term response and how these emerging devices are best deployed to ensure proper expansion. The challenge is to find ways to do so safely and efficiently as this complex optimization must ultimately happen in the context of patients who simply need to be treated.

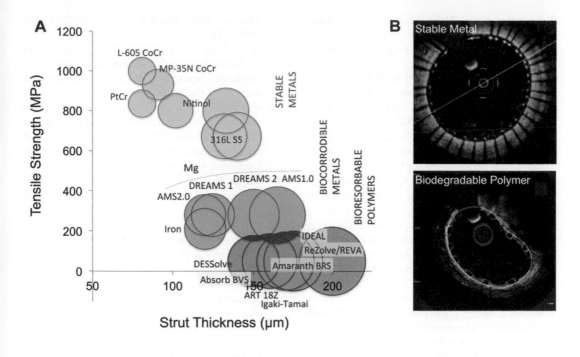

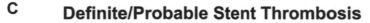

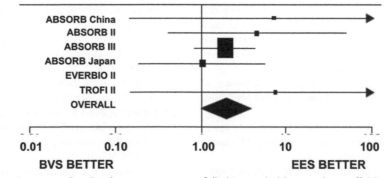

Fig. 6. Many strategies are under development to create fully bioresorbable vascular scaffolds (BVS), although there are interwoven design and material challenges. (A) Low strength materials require larger struts. As a class, stable metals (gray) are stronger than biocorrodible metals (magnesium, iron; blue), which are stronger than bioresorbable polymers (red). (B) Although stable metals provide excellent radial support, BVS performance requires further optimization as evidenced by the circular and elliptical cross-sections, respectively. (C) Initial clinical data suggest an increased risk of scaffold thrombosis with BVS. (Adapted from Cassese S, Byrne RA, Ndrepepa G, et al. Everolimus-eluting bioresorbable vascular scaffolds versus everolimus-eluting metallic stents: a meta-analysis of randomised controlled trials. Lancet 2015;387(10018):537–44; with permission.)

ACKNOWLEDGMENTS

We would like to thank Professor Elazer R. Edelman for insights and support in writing this review, as well as the Institute for Medical Engineering and Science Clinical Research Center (IMES/CRC) at the Massachusetts Institute of Technology for providing access to informational resources.

REFERENCES

1. Williams DF. On the mechanisms of biocompatibility. Biomaterials 2008;29:2941–53.
2. Kolandaivelu K, Edelman ER. Environmental influences on endovascular stent platelet reactivity: an in vitro comparison of stainless steel and gold surfaces. J Biomed Mater Res A 2004;70:186–93.

3. Sigwart U, Puel J, Mirkovitch V, et al. Intravascular stents to prevent occlusion and restenosis after transluminal angioplasty. N Engl J Med 1987;316: 701–6.

4. Byrne RA, Joner M, Kastrati A. Stent thrombosis and restenosis: what have we learned and where are we going? The Andreas Gruntzig Lecture ESC 2014. Eur Heart J 2015;36:3320–31.

5. Rogers C, Edelman ER. Endovascular stent design dictates experimental restenosis and thrombosis. Circulation 1995;91:2995–3001.

6. Alfonso F, Byrne RA, Rivero F, et al. Current treatment of in-stent restenosis. J Am Coll Cardiol 2014;63:2659–73.

7. Nakano M, Yahagi K, Otsuka F, et al. Causes of early stent thrombosis in patients presenting with acute coronary syndrome: an ex vivo human autopsy study. J Am Coll Cardiol 2014;63:2510–20.

8. Windecker S, Meier B. Late coronary stent thrombosis. Circulation 2007;116:1952–65.

9. Rogers C, Welt FG, Karnovsky MJ, et al. Monocyte recruitment and neointimal hyperplasia in rabbits. Coupled inhibitory effects of heparin. Arterioscler Thromb Vasc Biol 1996;16:1312–8.

10. Joner M, Finn AV, Farb A, et al. Pathology of drug-eluting stents in humans: delayed healing and late thrombotic risk. J Am Coll Cardiol 2006;48:193–202.

11. Finn AV, Joner M, Nakazawa G, et al. Pathological correlates of late drug-eluting stent thrombosis: strut coverage as a marker of endothelialization. Circulation 2007;115:2435–41.

12. Wu KK, Thiagarajan P. Role of endothelium in thrombosis and hemostasis. Annu Rev Med 1996; 47:315–31.

13. Sprague EA, Palmaz JC. A model system to assess key vascular responses to biomaterials. J Endovasc Ther 2005;12:594–604.

14. Nakamura S, Hall P, Gaglione A, et al. High pressure assisted coronary stent implantation accomplished without intravascular ultrasound guidance and subsequent anticoagulation. J Am Coll Cardiol 1997;29:21–7.

15. Serruys PW, de Jaegere P, Kiemeneij F, et al. A comparison of balloon-expandable-stent implantation with balloon angioplasty in patients with coronary artery disease. N Engl J Med 1994;331: 489–95.

16. Lowe HC, Oesterle SN, Khachigian LM. Coronary in-stent restenosis: current status and future strategies. J Am Coll Cardiol 2002;39:183–93.

17. O'Brien B, Carroll W. The evolution of cardiovascular stent materials and surfaces in response to clinical drivers: a review. Acta Biomater 2009;5: 945–58.

18. Nazneen F, Herzog G, Arrigan DWM, et al. Surface chemical and physical modification in stent technology for the treatment of coronary artery disease.

J Biomed Mater Res B Appl Biomater 2012;100B: 1989–2014.

19. Airoldi F, Colombo A, Tavano D, et al. Comparison of diamond-like carbon-coated stents versus uncoated stainless steel stents in coronary artery disease. Am J Cardiol 2004;93:474–7.

20. Antoniucci D, Valenti R, Migliorini A, et al. Clinical and angiographic outcomes following elective implantation of the Carbostent in patients at high risk of restenosis and target vessel failure. Catheter Cardiovasc Interv 2001;54:420–6.

21. Babapulle MN, Eisenberg MJ. Coated stents for the prevention of restenosis: Part II. Circulation 2002;106:2859–66.

22. Windecker S, Mayer I, De Pasquale G, et al. Stent coating with titanium-nitride-oxide for reduction of neointimal hyperplasia. Circulation 2001;104: 928–33.

23. Windecker S, Simon R, Lins M, et al. Randomized comparison of a titanium-nitride-oxide–coated stent with a stainless steel stent for coronary revascularization: the TiNOX trial. Circulation 2005;111: 2617–22.

24. Pilgrim T, Raber L, Limacher A, et al. Comparison of titanium-nitride-oxide-coated stents with zotarolimus-eluting stents for coronary revascularization a randomized controlled trial. JACC Cardiovasc Interv 2011;4: 672–82.

25. Mani G, Feldman MD, Patel D, et al. Coronary stents: A materials perspective. Biomaterials 2007; 28:1689–710.

26. Vadgama P. Surface biocompatibility. Annu Rep Prog Chem, Sect C: Phys Chem 2005;101:14–52.

27. Milleret V, Buzzi S, Gehrig P, et al. Protein adsorption steers blood contact activation on engineered cobalt chromium alloy oxide layers. Acta Biomater 2015;24:343–51.

28. Ruckenstein E, Gourisankar SV. A surface energetic criterion of blood compatibility of foreign surfaces. J Colloid Interface Sci 1984;101:436–51.

29. Haude M, Lee SWL, Worthley SG, et al. The REMEDEE Trial: a randomized comparison of a combination sirolimus-eluting endothelial progenitor cell capture stent with a paclitaxel-eluting stent. JACC Cardiovasc Interv 2013;6:334–43.

30. Hezi-Yamit A, Sullivan C, Wong J, et al. Impact of polymer hydrophilicity on biocompatibility: implication for DES polymer design. J Biomed Mater Res A 2009;90:133–41.

31. Zheng H, Barragan P, Corcos T, et al. Clinical experience with a new biocompatible phosphorylcholine-coated coronary stent. J Invasive Cardiol 1999;11: 608–14.

32. Abizaid A, Popma JJ, Tanajura LF, et al. Clinical and angiographic results of percutaneous coronary revascularization using a trilayer stainless steel-tantalum-stainless steel phosphorylcholine-coated

stent: the TriMaxx trial. Catheter Cardiovasc Interv 2007;70:914–9.

33. Atalar E, Haznedaroglu I, Aytemir K, et al. Effects of stent coating on platelets and endothelial cells after intracoronary stent implantation. Clin Cardiol 2001;24:159–64.

34. Denardo SJ, Carpinone PL, Vock DM, et al. Changes to polymer surface of drug-eluting stents during balloon expansion. JAMA 2012;307:2148–50.

35. Virmani R, Liistro F, Stankovic G, et al. Mechanism of late in-stent restenosis after implantation of a paclitaxel derivate-eluting polymer stent system in humans. Circulation 2002;106:2649–51.

36. Higuchi A, Sugiyama K, Yoon BO, et al. Serum protein adsorption and platelet adhesion on pluronic-adsorbed polysulfone membranes. Biomaterials 2003;24:3235–45.

37. Milleret V, Ziogas A, Buzzi S, et al. Effect of oxide layer modification of CoCr stent alloys on blood activation and endothelial behavior. J Biomed Mater Res B Appl Biomater 2015;103:629–40.

38. Li L, Mirhosseini N, Michael A, et al. Enhancement of endothelialisation of coronary stents by laser surface engineering. Lasers Surg Med 2013;45:608–16.

39. Wan P, Wu J, Tan L, et al. Research on super-hydrophobic surface of biodegradable magnesium alloys used for vascular stents. Mater Sci Eng C Mater Biol Appl 2013;33:2885–90.

40. Samaroo HD, Lu J, Webster TJ. Enhanced endothelial cell density on NiTi surfaces with sub-micron to nanometer roughness. Int J Nanomedicine 2008;3:75–82.

41. Ranjan A, Webster TJ. Increased endothelial cell adhesion and elongation on micron-patterned nano-rough poly(dimethylsiloxane) films. Nanotechnology 2009;20:305102.

42. Dibra A, Kastrati A, Mehilli J, et al. Influence of stent surface topography on the outcomes of patients undergoing coronary stenting: a randomized double-blind controlled trial. Catheter Cardiovasc Interv 2005;65:374–80.

43. Kolandaivelu K, Swaminathan R, Gibson WJ, et al. Stent thrombogenicity early in high-risk interventional settings is driven by stent design and deployment and protected by polymer-drug coatings. Circulation 2011;123:1400–9.

44. O'Brien CC, Lopes AC, Kolandaivelu K, et al. Vascular Response to Experimental Stent Malapposition and Under-Expansion. Ann Biomed Eng 2016. [Epub ahead of print].

45. Rikhtegar F, Wyss C, Stok KS, et al. Hemodynamics in coronary arteries with overlapping stents. J Biomech 2014;47:505–11.

46. Kastrati A, Mehilli J, Dirschinger J, et al. Intracoronary stenting and angiographic results: strut thickness effect on restenosis outcome (ISAR-STEREO) trial. Circulation 2001;103:2816–21.

47. Soucy NV, Feygin JM, Tunstall R, et al. Strut tissue coverage and endothelial cell coverage: a comparison between bare metal stent platforms and platinum chromium stents with and without everolimus-eluting coating. EuroIntervention 2010;6:630–7.

48. Bourantas CV, Papafaklis MI, Kotsia A, et al. Effect of the endothelial shear stress patterns on neointimal proliferation following drug-eluting bio-resorbable vascular scaffold implantation: an optical coherence tomography study. JACC Cardiovasc Interv 2014;7:315–24.

49. O'Brien CC, Kolandaivelu K, Brown J, et al. Constraining OCT with knowledge of device design enables high accuracy hemodynamic assessment of endovascular implants. PLoS One 2016;11(2):e0149178.

50. Yan BPY, Ajani AE, Waksman R. Drug-eluting stents for the treatment of in-stent restenosis: a clinical review. Cardiovasc Revasc Med 2005;6:38–43.

51. Hwang CW, Wu D, Edelman ER. Physiological transport forces govern drug distribution for stent-based delivery. Circulation 2001;104:600–5.

52. Creel CJ, Lovich MA, Edelman ER. Arterial paclitaxel distribution and deposition. Circ Res 2000; 86:879–84.

53. Artzi N, Tzafriri AR, Faucher KM, et al. Sustained efficacy and arterial drug retention by a fast drug eluting cross-linked fatty acid coronary stent coating. Ann Biomed Eng 2015;44(2):276–86.

54. Hezi-Yamit A, Sullivan C, Wong J, et al. Novel high-throughput polymer biocompatibility screening designed for SAR (structure-activity relationship): application for evaluating polymer coatings for cardiovascular drug-eluting stents. Comb Chem High Throughput Screen 2009;12:664–76.

55. Perkins LEL, Boeke-Purkis KH, Wang Q, et al. Xience V everolimus-eluting coronary stent system: a preclinical assessment. J Interv Cardiol 2009;22:s28–40.

56. Virmani R, Guagliumi G, Farb A, et al. Localized hypersensitivity and late coronary thrombosis secondary to a sirolimus-eluting stent: should we be cautious? Circulation 2004;109:701–5.

57. Pfisterer M, Brunner-La Rocca HP, Buser PT, et al. Late clinical events after clopidogrel discontinuation may limit the benefit of drug-eluting stents: an observational study of drug-eluting versus bare-metal stents. J Am Coll Cardiol 2006;48:2584–91.

58. Kolandaivelu K, Bhatt DL. Overcoming 'resistance' to antiplatelet therapy: targeting the issue of non-adherence. Nat Rev Cardiol 2010;7:461–7.

59. Guagliumi G, Ikejima H, Sirbu V, et al. Impact of drug release kinetics on vascular response to different zotarolimus-eluting stents implanted in patients with long coronary stenoses: the LongOCT study (Optical Coherence Tomography in Long Lesions). JACC Cardiovasc Interv 2011;4:778–85.

60. Joner M, Nakazawa G, Finn AV, et al. Endothelial cell recovery between comparator polymer-based

drug-eluting stents. J Am Coll Cardiol 2008;52: 333–42.

61. Bangalore S, Kumar S, Fusaro M, et al. Short- and long-term outcomes with drug-eluting and bare-metal coronary stents: a mixed-treatment comparison analysis of 117 762 patient-years of follow-up from randomized trials. Circulation 2012;125:2873–91.

62. Bangalore S, Amoroso N, Fusaro M, et al. Out- comes with various drug-eluting or bare metal stents in patients with ST-segment-elevation myocardial infarction: a mixed treatment compari- son analysis of trial level data from 34 068 patient-years of follow-up from randomized trials. Circ Cardiovasc Interv 2013;6:378–90.

63. Abizaid A, Costa JR Jr. New drug-eluting stents: an overview on biodegradable and polymer-free next- generation stent systems. Circ Cardiovasc Interv 2010;3:384–93.

64. Costa JR Jr, Abizaid A, Costa R, et al. 1-year results of the hydroxyapatite polymer-free sirolimus- eluting stent for the treatment of single de novo coronary lesions: the VESTASYNC I trial. JACC Car- diovasc Interv 2009;2:422–7.

65. Byrne RA, Iijima R, Mehilli J, et al. Durability of anti- restenotic efficacy in drug-eluting stents with and without permanent polymer. JACC Cardiovasc Interv 2009;2:291–9.

66. Bangalore S, Toklu B, Amoroso N, et al. Bare metal stents, durable polymer drug eluting stents, and biodegradable polymer drug eluting stents for cor- onary artery disease: mixed treatment comparison meta-analysis. BMJ 2013;347:f6625.

67. Kereiakes DJ, Meredith IT, Windecker S, et al. Effi- cacy and safety of a novel bioabsorbable polymer- coated, everolimus-eluting coronary stent: the EVOLVE II Randomized Trial. Circ Cardiovasc Interv 2015;8 [pii:e002372].

68. Vroman I, Tighzert L. Biodegradable polymers. Materials 2009;2:307–44.

69. Ferdous J, Kolachalama VB, Kolandaivelu K, et al. Degree of bioresorbable vascular scaffold

expansion modulates loss of essential function. Acta Biomater 2015;26:195–204.

70. Alexy RD, Levi DS. Materials and manufacturing technologies available for production of a pediatric bioabsorbable stent. Biomed Res Int 2013;2013: 137985.

71. Agrawal CM, Athanasiou KA. Technique to control pH in vicinity of biodegrading PLA-PGA implants. J Biomed Mater Res 1997;38:105–14.

72. Shazly T, Kolachalama VB, Ferdous J, et al. Assess- ment of material by-product fate from bioresorbable vascular scaffolds. Ann Biomed Eng 2012;40:955–65.

73. Stefanini GG, Byrne RA, Serruys PW, et al. Biode- gradable polymer drug-eluting stents reduce the risk of stent thrombosis at 4 years in patients under- going percutaneous coronary intervention: a pooled analysis of individual patient data from the ISAR-TEST 3, ISAR-TEST 4, and LEADERS ran- domized trials. Eur Heart J 2012;33:1214–22.

74. Otsuka F, Cheng Q, Yahagi K, et al. Acute thrombo- genicity of a durable polymer everolimus-eluting stent relative to contemporary drug-eluting stents with biodegradable polymer coatings assessed ex vivo in a swine shunt model. JACC Cardiovasc Interv 2015;8:1248–60.

75. Serruys PW, Garcia-Garcia HM, Onuma Y. From metallic cages to transient bioresorbable scaffolds: change in paradigm of coronary revascularization in the upcoming decade? Eur Heart J 2012;33:16–25.

76. Ormiston JA, Serruys PWS. Bioabsorbable coronary stents. Circ Cardiovasc Interv 2009;2:255–60.

77. Kawamoto H, Jabbour RJ, Tanaka A, et al. The bio- resorbable scaffold: will oversizing affect out- comes? JACC Cardiovasc Interv 2016;9:299–300.

78. Moravej M, Mantovani D. Biodegradable metals for cardiovascular stent application: interests and new opportunities. Int J Mol Sci 2011;12:4250–70.

79. Cassese S, Byrne RA, Ndrepepa G, et al. Everoli- mus-eluting bioresorbable vascular scaffolds versus everolimus-eluting metallic stents: a meta-analysis of randomised controlled trials. Lancet 2015; 387(10018):537–44.

Endovascular Drug Delivery and Drug Elution Systems: First Principles

Abraham Rami Tzafriri, PhD[a,b,*], Elazer Reuven Edelman, MD, PhD[b,c]

KEYWORDS

- Controlled release • Drug-eluting stents • Drug-filled stents • Polymer-free stents • Diffusion
- Dissolution • Distribution • Retention

KEY POINTS

- Because the effects of combination drug-eluting devices are multifactorial, designs abound and there is still room for innovation.
- Drug concentrations in tissues are predictive of effect and are not synonymous with delivered dose.
- Thus, although promising drug pharmacology is requisite, achieving adequate drug distribution and retention is key.
- Understanding and computationally modeling the determinants of drug release kinetics and tissue distribution can help further drive innovation at reduced cost.

INTRODUCTION

Endovascular drug-eluting stents (DESs) and more recently drug-eluting balloons, have revolutionized, and continue to revolutionize, the treatment of atherosclerosis in coronary and peripheral vasculature. The key has been to identify biologic agents that can counter the hyperplastic tissue responses to device expansion/implantation and to develop effective local delivery strategies that can maintain efficacious drug levels across the artery wall over the course of device effects (Fig. 1). This article reviews the various local drug delivery strategies implemented in approved and emerging endovascular devices, explains the mechanisms they use for drug release, and provides a mechanistic basis for relating drug release mode to arterial drug distribution and effect.

TISSUE PHARMACOKINETICS CAN LIMIT DRUG EFFICACY

Restenosis was recognized early as a clinical syndrome and a range of systemic pharmacologic therapies showed promise in vitro but failed in animals or humans. It became apparent (see Fig. 1) that the lesions to be combated were focal not diffuse and that systemic delivery not only exposed the great mass of unaffected tissues but diluted the desired target effects. Local therapy, once embraced, required a different mindset than other administration modes because issues of targeting, penetration, and retention now dominated rather than dosing. Administered dose is less important than these other forces, necessitating not simply a change in perspective but obviating qualitative, inferential approaches. The complexity of

Disclosure: A.R. Tzafriri is an employee of CBSET, a nonprofit contract research organization. E.R. Edelman is a paid consultant to Atrium/Maquet, MiCell Medical Technologies, and 480 Medical, and has sponsored research agreements with Boston Scientific and Medtronic.
Funding: This study was supported in part by grants from the NIH (RO1 GM-49039) to E.R. Edelman.
[a] Department of Applied Sciences, CBSET, Lexington, MA, USA; [b] IMES, MIT, 77 Massachusetts Avenue, Building E25-438, Cambridge, MA 02139, USA; [c] Division of Cardiovascular Medicine, Department of Medicine, Brigham and Women's Hospital, Harvard Medical School, 75 Francis Street, Boston, MA 02115, USA
* Corresponding author. Department of Applied Sciences, CBSET, Lexington, MA.
E-mail address: rtzafriri@cbset.org

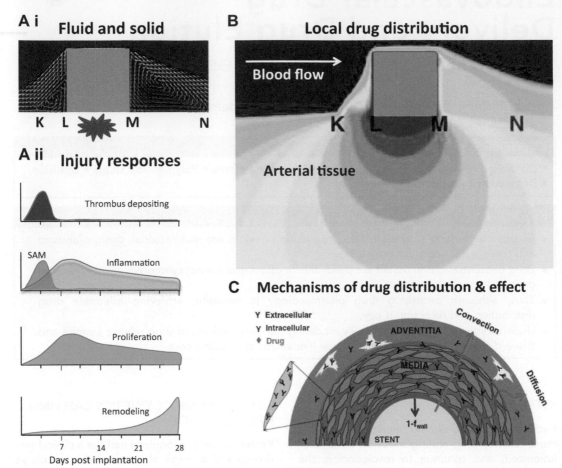

A i   Fluid and solid

K L M N

A ii   Injury responses

Thrombus depositing

SAM   Inflammation

Proliferation

Remodeling

7   14   21   28
Days post implantation

B   Local drug distribution

Blood flow

K L M N

Arterial tissue

C   Mechanisms of drug distribution & effect

Y Extracellular
Y Intracellular
♦ Drug

Convection

ADVENTITIA

MEDIA

Diffusion

$1-f_{wall}$

STENT

Fig. 1. Endovascular drug delivery occurs in the context of tissue response to mechanical forces. (A.i) Stent implantation mechanically injures the arterial wall and induces strut-proximal (K-L) and strut-distal (M-N) recirculation zones. (A.ii) This process triggers 4 phases of vascular repair: platelet-rich thrombus accumulates at areas of deep strut injury, accounting for most early luminal loss. Coincident with thrombus deposition, inflammatory cells, predominantly surface-adherent monocytes (SAM), are recruited to the injury site, both at and between the struts, before migrating into the neointima as tissue-infiltrating monocytes. Proliferation of smooth muscle cells and monocyte/macrophages within the neointima peaks at 7 days after implantation and continues at greater than baseline levels for weeks thereafter. Collagen deposition in the adventitia and throughout the tunica media and neointima leads to arterial shrinkage, or remodeling, causing compression of the artery on the stent struts from without. (B) Model predicted drug distribution surrounding the square strut depicted in A.i. Maximal concentrations (*red*) occur immediately beneath the strut, minimal concentrations (*blue*) occur between struts. (C) Depiction of the processes governing arterial drug distribution and effect: transmural drug convection along a pressure gradient, diffusion driven by concentration gradients, drug binding to nonspecific binding tissue proteins and intracellular receptors. (*Adapted from [A.i, B]* Kolachalama VB, Levine EG, Edelman ER. Luminal flow amplifies stent-based drug deposition in arterial bifurcations. PLoS One 2009;4:e8105, with permission; and [A.ii] Edelman ER, Rogers C. Pathobiologic responses to stenting. Am J Cardiol 1998;81:6E, with permission; and *Reproduced from [C]* Tzafriri AR, Groothuis A, Price GS, et al. Stent elution rate determines drug deposition and receptor-mediated effects. J Control Release 2012;161:920, with permission.)

the issues required experimental and computational modeling analyses, which created a quantitative framework by which to evaluate temporal and spatial extents of drug distribution in the arterial wall and correlate patterns with successful tissue effects (**Fig. 2**).

The challenge of optimizing local delivery increases dramatically given the innovations and complexity in modern stent designs, because tissue distribution after stent delivery tends to mirror stent coating geometry (see **Fig. 2A**). Different designs differentially affect luminal washout relative to drug diffusion in the tissue, and can result in peak drug concentrations and toxicity immediately adjacent to stent struts (see **Fig. 2B**). The disparity between peak and

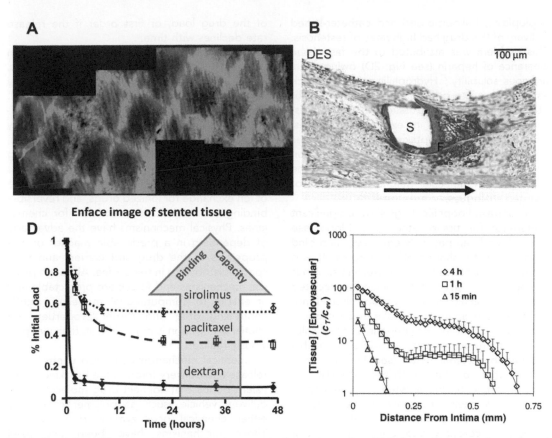

Fig. 2. Local drug efficacy can be limited by drug penetration and retention. (A) Enface microscopy of stent-based delivery of fluorescein mirrors stet geometry. Depicts fluorescent microscopy (visualizing the model drug fluorescein). (B) Maximal drug deposition occurs immediately beneath the strut, although distal recirculation zones can also deposit high drug concentrations as shown by fibrin deposition 28 days after implantation of paclitaxel-eluting stents. Carstair's fibrin stain. (C) Uniform endovascular drug delivery only saturates the artery wall after sufficiently prolonged exposures. Thus, although the 15-minute luminal exposure to paclitaxel results in an intimal drug concentration greater than 10-fold higher than in the luminal infusate, the arterial media is devoid of drug. (D) Fractional drug retention by presaturated arteries scales with the tissue's binding capacity for the drug. F, fibrin; S, strut. [A] From Hwang CW, Wu D, Edelman ER. Physiological transport forces govern drug distribution for stent-based delivery. Circulation 2001;104:600–5; with permission; [B] From Balakrishnan B, Tzafriri AR, Seifert P, et al. Strut position, blood flow, and drug deposition: implications for single and overlapping drug-eluting stents. Circulation 2005;111:2958–65; with permission; [C] From Creel CJ, Lovich MA, Edelman ER. Arterial paclitaxel distribution and deposition. Circ Res 2000;86:879–84; with permission; and Adapted from [D] Levin AD, Vukmirovic N, Hwang CW, et al. Specific binding to intracellular proteins determines arterial transport properties for rapamycin and paclitaxel. Proc Natl Acad Sci U S A 2004;101:9465, with permission.)

trough drug concentrations can be reduced by altering the rate of drug elution[1] or through engineering of strut shape to increase the spatial extent and drug delivery role of strut-distal recirculation zones[2] but this requires a sophisticated perspective (see Fig. 1B). As reviewed later, stent-based delivery can be rendered more uniform by intentionally varying drug loading along the device surface or through deployment of drug-loaded coating or particles to interstrut zones.[3,4]

Notably, even uniform endovascular drug delivery does not ensure adequate transmural drug distribution unless the duration of delivery is sufficiently long (see Fig. 2C). The minimal duration for adequate arterial distribution increases with endothelial integrity and resistance to drug absorption, and tends to be higher for larger drugs that show lower tissue diffusivities and higher steric retardation, although drug charge and lipophilicity are also important factors.[5,6]

Moreover, even when drug saturates the artery wall, drug clearance can render the therapy inefficacious. Thus, for example, although heparin pharmacology is well suited to countering the acute and sustained vascular responses to angioplasty, balloon-based and catheter-based delivery of this drug had high rates of restenosis. This problem was attributed to the fast tissue clearance of heparin (see Fig. 2D) owing to its aqueous solubility.[7] Hydrophilic molecules such as heparin have a greater propensity for distributing into blood than into tissue, and within the tissue tend to reside in extracellular spaces. Consequently, tissue uptake and clearance rates of soluble drugs tend to scale with their diffusion coefficients and can be prolonged through the use of high-molecular-weight analogues or charged analogues.

In contrast, lipophilic drugs show a significant preference for tissue rather than blood (see Fig. 2C) and can passively enter cells and bind to high-affinity pharmacologic targets. It was not until compounds like paclitaxel and sirolimus analogues were used that clinicians appreciated that there was also a need for local tissue binding to ensure adequate uptake and retention. These drugs, smaller than heparin and less soluble than many compounds, are more sustainably retained by arterial tissue (see Fig. 2D) in a manner that correlates with the expression of drug bindings sites in the tissue[6,8]; these properties underlie their emergence as the drugs of choice for stent-based and balloon-based delivery in coronary and peripheral vascular beds. Importantly, drug distribution and retention are not solely determined by the mode of delivery and the properties of the drug, and also depend on tissue morphology because different ultrastructural tissue elements can show disparate resistance and capacitance for the same drug.[9,10]

MECHANISMS CONTROLLING LOCAL DRUG RELEASE

As described earlier, duration of drug exposure affects the extent of arterial distribution and retention and therefore the resulting biological effects of endovascular drug delivery. Thus, strategies for controlling drug dose and release kinetics have played an important role in endovascular drug delivery. In lieu of additional controlling factors, drug that is coated onto device surfaces tends to elute in a burst fashion, potentially overdosing the local tissue environment without sustaining efficacious levels. Although many DESs show some level of burst release, a significant fraction of the drug load is typically eluted in a sustained manner. The sustained elution component can vary between DESs, and are broadly classified as zero order if the rate of release is near constant until depletion

of the drug load, or first order if the release rate declines with time.

Despite the abundance of DES and balloon designs developed over the last 3 decades, only a few distinct physical mechanisms have been used to control drug release (Table 1). These mechanisms include diffusion of drug molecules along concentration gradients (usually through a rate-limiting polymer material layer), dissolution of the drug particles within a coating or within the tissue, dissolution and hydrolytic degradation of rate-limiting polymer layers, use of ion exchange for ionized drugs, and reversible binding to immobilized antibodies for chemokines. Physical mechanisms have the advantage of depending in a predictable manner on the properties of the drug and carriers and their spatial distribution in the device. Although physical mechanisms and forces are predictable and amenable to computational modeling, tightly controlling drug and carrier properties and spatial distribution is more difficult than was previously realized.[11,12]

Chemical mechanisms can also control drug release and delivery through the breaking of covalent bonds that connect drug molecules to a delivery vehicle, such as polymer chains, by either chemical or enzymatic degradation.[13] These mechanisms have been underused because of the need to chemically modify drugs for grafting to the delivery vehicle. Such modifications result in new chemical entities called prodrugs, adding regulatory scrutiny to previously approved drugs.

DEVICE-BASED ENDOVASCULAR DRUG DELIVERY STRATEGIES

Durable Adherent Coatings

First-generation and second-generation DESs used durable polymer coatings to adhere therapeutic drug loads to the stent and release it in diffusion-controlled manner. Such diffusion-controlled devices are broadly classified as matrix type or reservoir type (Fig. 3A, B). In matrix-type devices, such as the paclitaxel-eluting Taxus stent and the zotarolimus-eluting Endeavor stent, drug is released from the polymer matrix directly into the environment. For this reason, matrix devices are also referred to as monolithic devices. By contrast, reservoir-type devices such as the sirolimus-eluting Cypher stent and the everolimus-eluting Xience stent use at least 2 distinct layers, an internal drug reservoir and a thin external polymer layer, designed to limit the rate of drug elution from the internal drug reservoir. Hybrid multilayer coating designs

Table 1
Popular mechanisms for controlling endovascular drug release

Mechanism	Schematic	Conditions	Design Parameters
Diffusion		Drug must be mobile within coating or reservoir	Drug size, lipophilicity, loading gradient, polymer composition, and molecular weight
Dissolution		Solid drug particles must dissolve before drug diffusion	Drug particle size and solubility, reservoir volume, water accessibility
Erosion		Polymer erosion increases the mobility of trapped drug	Polymer type, molecular weight, and glass transition temperature; drug size and lipophilicity
Ion exchange		Charged drug, oppositely charged device-surface groups	Ratio of drug load to surface charge density
Antibody binding		Drug binds to device-surface epitopes	Ratio of drug load to surface binding sites

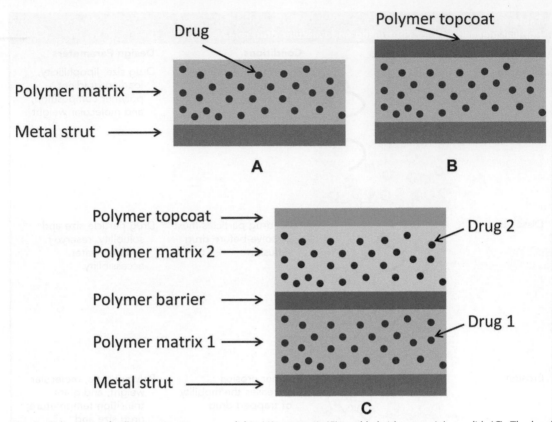

Fig. 3. Side views of adherent coatings: monolithic (*A*), reservoir (*B*), and hybrid reservoir/monolith (*C*). The local drug efficacy can be limited by drug penetration and retention.

(Fig. 3C) have also been developed as a means of providing greater control over the release of 1 or more drugs, while optimizing acute and sustained biocompatibility.[13]

In theory, drug release from durable-coated DES designs can be predictably controlled based on the designed thicknesses of the polymer and drug layers and the concepts of diffusion and dissolution. However, multiple rounds of spray coating can lead to considerable mixing between sequential layers[12] and to enrichment of drug near the surface.[14] Thus, although the Cypher stent was designed as a reservoir-type DES,[13] imaging reveals drug presence in the external rate-limiting polymer layer, resulting in monolithic-type diffusion-controlled release.[15] Because spray coating is traditionally applied to stents that are mounted to a spinning mandrel, this technique also limits control over spatial drug coating design. Thus, it is difficult to optimize interstrut drug delivery via enrichment of luminal and distal coating, or to coat different drugs on the abluminal and luminal aspects of stents for inhibiting restenosis while promoting endothelialization. More sophisticated inkjet and microdrop injection

technologies can provide better-controlled spatial coating design at the micro and macro levels.[16] In addition, layer-by-layer assembly of polyelectrolytes is a promising strategy for high-fidelity engineering of device surfaces and ion-exchange controlled release of charged biologic agents such as DNA and small interfering RNA.[13]

Application of the spray iterations to static flat metal sheets can overcome the limitations seen with spray application to spinning stents. Such a procedure allows shorter spray run times but longer dry times and therefore minimal mixing between successive layers. Moreover, en face spraying onto a static sheet is ideally suited for high-fidelity abluminal coating and can be programmed to provide controlled heterogeneous coatings. The authors recently showed that en face spray coating of flat cobalt-chromium sheets with tightly controlled concentrations of the drug ridaforolimus and 2 polymer types provided monolithic and hybrid reservoir/monolithic-type coatings. Drug release from these DES was well predicted by a diffusion-based model that accounts for the predetermined layer thicknesses and compositions and a composition-dependent diffusion coefficient.[17] Such a combination of tightly controlled spray coating and computational modeling provides truly customizable release kinetics.

Biodegradable Adherent Coatings

Concern for persistent adverse responses to durable polymeric coatings prompted the development of more biocompatible durable polymeric materials or bioerodible coatings that are absorbed over the course of stent implantation.[18] Some designs sought to minimize polymer-tissue contact by incorporating polymer/drug formulations into sculpted surface inlays in the form of grooves and holes available on the struts using microdispensers.[13,18] The grooves and holes vary in size, shape, and location relative to the struts and can incorporate the polymer in monolithic, reservoir, or hybrid reservoir/monolithic design. In contrast, other clinicians attributed the persistence of safety concerns with durable-coated metallic stents to the persistence of the metallic scaffold long after acute responses and drug delivery have ceased, providing an impetus for the use of biodegradable polymeric scaffolds as vascular mechanical supports and drug delivery platforms.[18]

Despite the abundance of biodegradable DESs and scaffold designs, the optimum temporal balancing of erosion and drug release still awaits full definition because most erodible scaffolds and stents with erodible coatings release their entire drug load before erosion (Fig. 4), maintaining diffusion-limited release kinetics similar to durable-coated DESs[15] but also necessarily prolonging the duration of any adverse polymer effects. Because of the notion that restenosis inhibition by sirolimus analogues requires sustained delivery, the duration of drug release from biodegradable coatings and scaffolds is typically comparable with that of first-generation Cypher stents (see Fig. 4). This misguided focus on release kinetics as a driver of effect, rather than tissue retention, has restricted the choice of DES coating materials. In particular, natural bioerodible polymers that permeabilize quickly during hydrolysis and absorption have been shunned in favor of synthetic polymers that are absorbed over the course of several months[18]; for example, polylactic acid, polyglycolic acid, copolymer, or other variations thereof (see Fig. 4). These synthetic materials may produce local irritation caused by the release of acidic degradation products, can delay healing, and may transiently place the artery at increased risk of adverse reaction.[19]

The authors hypothesized that naturally derived coating compositions that degrade rapidly can deliver controlled volumes of drug without loss of biological effect and at reduced periods of tissue vulnerability. To examine this hypothesis, cobalt-chromium stents were conformally coated with a novel cross-linked omega-3 fatty acid (O3FA)–based coating[20] that is 85% absorbed (Fig. 5A) and elutes 97% of its sirolimus analogue (corolimus) load within 8 days of implantation (Fig. 5B). Evaluation in pig coronary arteries revealed sustained efficacious drug levels that were similar to those achieved by slow-eluting durable-coated sirolimus-eluting stents (Fig. 5C) and resulted in superior efficacy and more benign tissue response. Computational modeling confirmed that corolimus distributes in arterial tissue with the same diffusion and binding constants as sirolimus and explained that its sustained retention after fast elution from the O3FA DES was facilitated by high-affinity binding of drug to intracellular FKBP12 (see Fig. 5C). The same computational model predicts that corolimus saturates greater than 65% up to 8 days after implantation and that the dissociation of the drug-FKBP12 complex linearly tracks with coating absorption (Fig. 5D). Thus, late coating absorption and drug inhibitory effects decline in a linearly parallel manner, suggesting that the former drives the latter, and representing a new paradigm in stent-based drug delivery. Clinical data suggest that late lumen loss has already stabilized after 6 months in the presence of O3FA (Cinatra DES) and continues to increase with the Cypher stent,[20] supporting the clinical validity of the O3FA DES product design approach.

Thus, tissue retention of sirolimus analogues can be achieved even with fast-elution kinetics following rapid coating erosion, with computational modeling identifying binding to tissue receptors as the mechanism of prolonged retention.[20] The composition of drug-eluting coatings can then be designed for optimal biocompatibility and bioabsorption rather than predominantly for sustained drug elution kinetics. This paradigm shift creates an opportunity for the use of a range of biocompatible materials that may have not otherwise have been considered.

Deployable Coatings

The DES designs highlighted earlier use durable and erodible coatings as stent adherent conduits for drug elution. By contrast, the absorbable r poly(lactic-co-glycolic acid) coating of the MiStent sirolimus-eluting stent is designed to soften

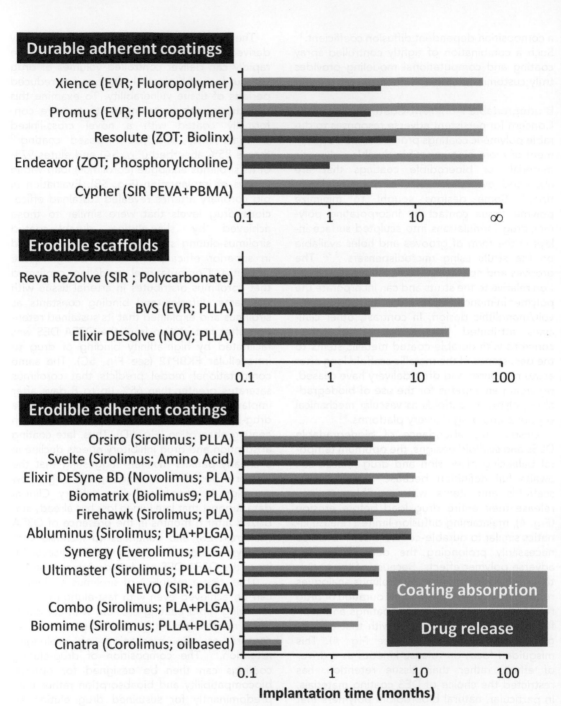

Fig. 4. Durations of drug release and coating absorption for a range of sirolimus analogue–eluting stents. CL, caprolactone; EVR, everolimus; NOV, Novolimus; SIR, sirolimus; ZOT, zotarolimus. (*Data from* Refs.[4,18,20,30,31])

and spread into the neointima by tissue remodeling forces (**Fig. 6**A) while carrying along its microcrystalline sirolimus load.[3] These intratissue polymer-encapsulated microcrystalline drug particles act as sustained drug delivery microdepots (microreservoirs) that ensure high tissue contents long after the stent has reverted to the bare metal state (**Fig. 6**B). By the same

token, during neointimal growth, the area of drug delivery increases dynamically beyond the immediate vicinity of the struts. Computational modeling showed that spread of coating to interstrut regions improves drug delivery to these areas and decreases gradients in drug distribution (**Fig. 6**C). At small migration distances, drug deposition near the struts may increase

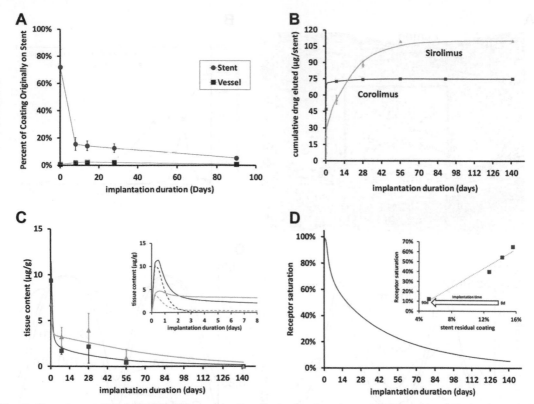

Fig. 5. Receptor-mediated sustained tissue retention. In vivo coating absorption (*A*) and local tissue pharmacokinetics (*B–D*) of a fast eluting O3FA DES. The O3FA coating quickly elutes off the stent with low accumulation in arterial tissue (*A*). This process results in faster release of corolimus from O3FA DES (*red*) compared with sirolimus release from Cypher Select Plus DES (*green*) in the same cohort (*B*). In vivo tissue contents (*symbols*) for both DESs are comparable tissue levels up to 56 days after implantation and closely predicted by a computational model that accounts for high-affinity drug binding to FKBP12 (*lines*). The inset shows that modeling that does not account for high-affinity drug binding to FKBP12 (*dashes*) predicts unrealistically fast tissue clearance. (*D*) Model predicted FKBP12 saturation by corolimus (*red line*) correlates linearly with in vivo coating absorption (*insert*). (*Reproduced from [A–C] Artzi N, Tzafriri AR, Faucher KM et al. Sustained efficacy and arterial drug retention by a fast drug eluting cross-linked fatty acid coronary stent coating. Ann Biomed Eng 2016;44(2):281–2; with permission.*)

because the greater surface area of elution can compensate for the decline in strut adherent coating. However, beyond a threshold distance (~100 μm), migration can appreciably decrease near-strut drug deposition (see **Fig. 6**C). Peak-trough levels 150 μm into the media were predicted to decline at a near constant rate of 1.7 ng/mg per 100-μm coating migration, reaching unity as the coating migrates ~0.5 mm distal to the strut.[21]

Whether or not the more homogeneous drug delivery provided by tissue deployed coatings comes at the expense of suboptimal dosing cannot be determined from total drug levels and requires insight into the concentration of therapeutically active drug that is bound to its intracellular target. Although labeling of a drug may enable tracking of total drug concentration

gradients, resolution of the concentration of sirolimus bound to FKBP12 was only possible through computational modeling (**Fig. 6**D). Such simulations predicted greater than or equal to 80% saturation of FKBP12 by drug, even in arteries in which coating remains fully conformal to the stent. However, although conformal stents bind 15% more receptors near than between struts, deployed coatings saturate 94% to 96% of receptors throughout the neointima (see **Fig. 6**D).

The novel insights provided by these studies are relevant to the expanding class of endovascular delivery devices that deliver drug in microcrystalline form, including drug-coated balloons and nanopolymer-coated[4] stents and balloons. Quantitative experimental and computational analyses of these devices have yet to be published.

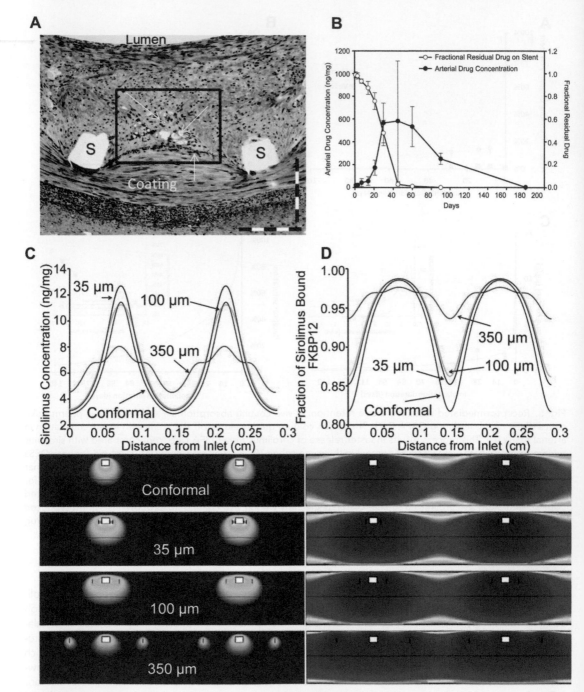

Fig. 6. Enhanced drug delivery capabilities from stents coated with absorbable polymer and crystalline drug. (*A*) Histopathology at 30 days identified coating as the negative image of space-occupying mass (*arrows*) between struts (*S*). Hematoxylin and eosin stain. (*B*) Drug release is complete within 45 to 60 days after stent implantation, but tissue levels remain at near peak levels long after. (*C*, *D*) Computational modeling predicted drug (*C*) and receptor binding (*D*) distribution patterns around a strut pair that is fully coated (conformal) or where the bottom coating deployed 35, 100, or 400 μm into interstrut zones. (*Reproduced from* Carlyle WC, McClain JB, Tzafriri AR, et al. Enhanced drug delivery capabilities from stents coated with absorbable polymer and crystalline drug. J Control Release 2012;162:564–5; with permission.)

Polymer-free Coated Stents

Some metallic DES designs dispense with polymer coatings, offering the potential advantages of avoiding long-term polymer material–induced hypersensitivity and potential thrombogenicity that necessitate long-term dual antiplatelet therapy, and alleviating concerns for coating peeling and cracking.[4,18,22] First-generation polymer-free stents (PFSs) were dip coated in ethanolic paclitaxel and did not meet the predetermined primary clinical end point of target vessel failure and the secondary end point of binary restenosis.[13] Preclinical evaluation of these dip-coated stents showed that most of the drug loss occurred before stent expansion and deployment,[13] and prompted the development of several different techniques for controlled drug elution from stents in the absence of a polymer[23] (Fig. 7A):

1. Direct attachment of drug to the stent surface using covalent bonding, or crystallization chemical precipitation on the stent surface.
2. Dissolving of the drug in a nonpolymeric biodegradable carrier on the stent surface.
3. Impregnation of the drug into surface micropores or nanopores formed by mechanical or electrochemical treatment of metallic surfaces, or on specialized inorganic surface coating.
4. Microinjection of the pure drug or drug formulated with nonpolymeric excipients into sculpted surface inlays or slots.

Similar to drug-coated balloons, second-generation PFSs rely on nondiffusive mechanisms, most commonly slow dissolution of sparsely soluble crystalline drug forms, to compensate for the absence of the tempering effects of a polymeric layer. This reliance has again focused attention on hydrophobic drugs, mostly on paclitaxel and sirolimus analogues because of their well-characterized antirestenotic pharmacologic effects, favorable tissue distribution, and retention properties. Clinical experience with second-generation PFSs has been promising, with several coronary PFSs receiving the CE (Conformité Européene) mark and the paclitaxel-eluting peripheral PFS receiving US Food and Drug Administration approval. Because of the differences in the eluted drugs, stent geometries, strut thicknesses, and surface morphologies, as well as the paucity of in vivo drug release data, the optimal kinetics of drug elution from PFSs have yet to be defined.

Preliminary insight into the dependence of PFS efficacy on sirolimus analogue release kinetics can be gained by contrasting the available tissue delivery profiles of these devices with efficacious bioresorbable-coated and durable-coated sirolimus DESs (Fig. 8). For example, the Yukon PFS elutes 66.4% and 85.5% of sirolimus loaded into its microporous surface within 7 and 21 days of in vitro deployment in a buffer solution.[24,25] During the first week of implantation, tissue concentrations provided by Yukon PFS exceed those provide by slow-eluting Cypher stents, but this is reversed by 10 days following a greater than 95% decline in tissue levels for the PFS (see Fig. 8). Incorporation of a biodegradable polymer along with sirolimus into the

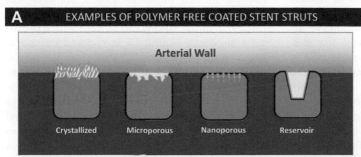

Fig. 7. Various polymer-free DES types. (A) Drug coated stent struts. (B) Drug filled stent strut.

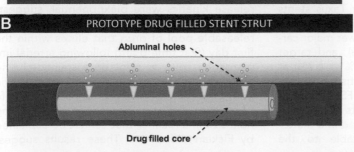

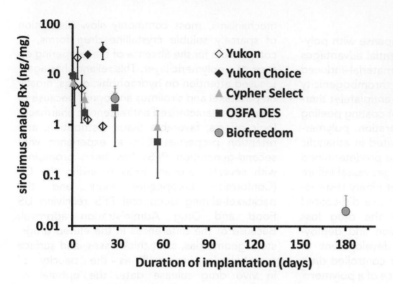

Fig. 8. Tissue concentrations achieved by sirolimus analogue–eluting PFS, and durable and bioerodible coated DES.[20,24,25,27] O3FA DES and Cypher Select data are from Fig. 5C.

microporous surface results in the Yukon Choice stent, which releases sirolimus at a near-constant rate during 28-day deployments in phosphate-buffered saline, and sustains high tissue levels up to 20 days after implantation (see Fig. 8). Clinical late lumen loss in de novo coronary lesions scaled with the duration of tissue retention, because Yukon PFS but not Yukon Choice was inferior to durable-coated Cypher stents.[26]

These clinical findings also scale with the relative duration of Sirolimus release from the 2 microporous stents. By contrast, clinical responses to the Biofreedom PFS, which elutes the extremely lipophilic Sirolimus analog Biolimus A9, scale with local tissue concentrations rather than released dose. Thus, although the Biofreedom PFS has been reported to release ~90% and ~99.9% by 2 and 28 days,[23,27] the associated tissue concentration in porcine arteries at 28 days[27] is comparable with that sustained by slower eluting durable-coated DESs (see Fig. 8). Similar to our findings with the fast-eluting O3FA-coated DES,[20] Biofreedom PFS showed reduced inflammation and wall thickening compared with the slower eluting durable-coated Cypher stents at 28 and 180 days.[27] Moreover, randomized clinical comparisons of Biofreedom PFS with Taxus stents found noninferior late lumen loss at 1 year (0.17 vs 0.35 mm), significantly lower major cardiac event rates (6.8% vs 10.0%), and target lesion revascularization rates (3.4% vs 6.7%) at 2 years.[22] In light of the sustained tissue concentration achieved by Biofreedom PFS, such positive preclinical and clinical results for a stent that releases ~90% of its drug load in a matter of 2 days are likely attributable to the

pharmacokinetic profile of the eluted drug. In particular, Tada and colleagues[27] highlighted that the extreme lipophilicity of Biolimus A9 relative to other sirolimus analogues endows it with more favorable tissue absorption and cell uptake. This plausible assertion should be investigated further using animal and computational models.

Drug-filled Stents

Drug-filled stents (DFSs) are a new class of a polymer-free DES technology currently being developed (Medtronic). In this design, the stent struts have a tubular configuration, with a hollow core; small access holes connect the inner core to the abluminal surface. Drug is loaded in the inner core and diffuses out through the holes into the vessel wall (Fig. 7B). Initial 90-day pig studies with a prototype sirolimus-eluting DFSs showed comparable drug release rates and tissue concentrations with the slow-eluting durable-coated Resolute stent and effective suppression of neointimal hyperplasia at 28 days compared with bare metal stents, with minimal inflammation through 90 days.[28] Follow-up analysis of the data revealed that sirolimus release kinetics were biexponential, suggesting the existence of an easily available and releasable pool of drug that elutes within the first day (first time point) following arterial implantation, plus a pool of sustained-eluting drug with a half-life of 28 to 32 days.[29] The pool of sustained-eluting drug and its half-life of release both decreased with increasing hole size in a manner that cannot be explained by Fickian diffusion.[29] These results suggest that drug-release kinetics from DFSs are predominantly dissolution controlled and can be modulating by altering hole size. Modeling analysis of this system is underway.

SUMMARY/DISCUSSION

Although endovascular drug delivery is now a mature field, the last few years have heralded a resurgence of innovation designed to improve performance and reduce cost. Every tenet of first-generation DESs has been reexamined and questioned, from the need for a persistent metallic scaffold, through the need for an adherent polymer coating as a drug-release reservoir, to the need for sustaining drug release. Although some clinicians call for the abolition of the polymer coating, others have expanded its role into a deployable carrier of crystalline drug. This article reviews the mechanistic basis underlying these technological innovations and discusses the critical role that quantitative experiments and computational modeling have played so far. These techniques are critical for understanding the interplay between device design, drug release, tissue distribution, and effect, and offer a powerful framework for further innovation.

REFERENCES

1. Balakrishnan B, Dooley JF, Kopia G, et al. Intravascular drug release kinetics dictate arterial drug deposition, retention, and distribution. J Control Release 2007;123:100–8.
2. Kolachalama VB, Tzafriri AR, Arifin DY, et al. Luminal flow patterns dictate arterial drug deposition in stent-based delivery. J Control Release 2009;133:24–30.
3. Carlyle WC, McClain JB, Tzafriri AR, et al. Enhanced drug delivery capabilities from stents coated with absorbable polymer and crystalline drug. J Control Release 2012;162:561–7.
4. Garg S, Bourantas C, Serruys PW. New concepts in the design of drug-eluting coronary stents. Nat Rev Cardiol 2013;10:248–60.
5. Hwang CW, Wu D, Edelman ER. Impact of transport and drug properties on the local pharmacology of drug-eluting stents. Int J Cardiovasc Intervent 2003;5:7–12.
6. Tzafriri AR, Levin AD, Edelman ER. Diffusion-limited binding explains binary dose response for local arterial and tumour drug delivery. Cell Prolif 2009; 42:348–63.
7. Lovich MA, Edelman ER. Computational simulations of local vascular heparin deposition and distribution. Am J Physiol 1996;271:H2014–24.
8. Levin AD, Vukmirovic N, Hwang CW, et al. Specific binding to intracellular proteins determines arterial transport properties for rapamycin and paclitaxel. Proc Natl Acad Sci U S A 2004;101:9463–7.
9. Hwang CW, Edelman ER. Arterial ultrastructure influences transport of locally delivered drugs. Circ Res 2002;90:826–32.
10. Hwang CW, Levin AD, Jonas M, et al. Thrombosis modulates arterial drug distribution for drug-eluting stents. Circulation 2005;111:1619–26.
11. Saylor DM, Guyer JE, Wheeler D, et al. Predicting microstructure development during casting of drug-eluting coatings. Acta Biomater 2011;7:604–13.
12. Balss KM, Llanos G, Papandreou G, et al. Quantitative spatial distribution of sirolimus and polymers in drug-eluting stents using confocal Raman microscopy. J Biomed Mater Res A 2008;85:258–70.
13. Acharya G, Park K. Mechanisms of controlled drug release from drug-eluting stents. Adv Drug Deliv Rev 2006;58:387–401.
14. Belu A, Mahoney C, Wormuth K. Chemical imaging of drug eluting coatings: combining surface analysis and confocal Raman microscopy. J Control Release 2008;126:111–21.
15. Tzafriri AR, Groothuis A, Price GS, et al. Stent elution rate determines drug deposition and receptor-mediated effects. J Control Release 2012;161:918–26.
16. Tarcha PJ, Verlee D, Hui HW, et al. The application of ink-jet technology for the coating and loading of drug-eluting stents. Ann Biomed Eng 2007;35:1791–9.
17. Tzafriri AR, Markham PM, LaRochelle AW, et al. CRT-500.10 ridaforolimus eluting stents with customizable diffusion controlled release kinetics and tissue uptake. JACC Cardiovasc Interventions 2016;9:S56.
18. Garg S, Serruys PW. Coronary stents: looking forward. J Am Coll Cardiol 2010;56:S43–78.
19. Shazly T, Kolachalama VB, Ferdous J, et al. Assessment of material by-product fate from bioresorbable vascular scaffolds. Ann Biomed Eng 2012;40:955–65.
20. Artzi N, Tzafriri AR, Faucher KM, et al. Sustained efficacy and arterial drug retention by a fast drug eluting cross-linked fatty acid coronary stent coating. Ann Biomed Eng 2016;44(2):276–86.
21. Tzafriri AR, Bailey L, Stanley J, et al. TCT-570 stents with absorbable tissue-deployable coatings can distribute drug more uniformly between struts. JACC 2012;60:B166.
22. Urban P, Abizaid A, Chevalier B, et al. Rationale and design of the LEADERS FREE trial: A randomized double-blind comparison of the BioFreedom drug-coated stent vs the Gazelle bare metal stent in patients at high bleeding risk using a short (1 month) course of dual antiplatelet therapy. Am Heart J 2013;165:704–9.

23. Chen W, Habraken TC, Hennink WE, et al. Polymer-free drug-eluting stents: an overview of coating strategies and comparison with polymer-coated drug-eluting stents. Bioconjug Chem 2015;26: 1277–88.

24. Steigerwald K, Merl S, Kastrati A, et al. The preclinical assessment of rapamycin-eluting, durable polymer-free stent coating concepts. Biomaterials 2009;30:632–7.

25. Wessely R, Hausleiter J, Michaelis C, et al. Inhibition of neointima formation by a novel drug-eluting stent system that allows for dose-adjustable, multiple, and on-site stent coating. Arterioscler Thromb Vasc Biol 2005;25:748–53.

26. Mehilli J, Byrne RA, Wieczorek A, et al. Randomized trial of three rapamycin-eluting stents with different coating strategies for the reduction of coronary restenosis. Eur Heart J 2008;29:1975–82.

27. Tada N, Virmani R, Grant G, et al. Polymer-free Biolimus A9-coated stent demonstrates more sustained intimal inhibition, improved healing, and reduced inflammation compared with a polymer-coated sirolimus-eluting cypher stent in a porcine model. Circ Cardiovasc Interv 2010;3: 174–83.

28. Stone G, Kirtane A, Abizaid A, et al. Preclinical results with a novel internally loaded drug -filled coronary stent. JACC 2015;65:A1762.

29. Tzafriri AR, Markham PM, Goshgarian J, et al. TCT-554 titratable drug delivery from drug filled stents. J Am Coll Cardiol 2015;66:B224–5.

30. Parker T, Dave V, Falotico R. Polymers for drug eluting stents. Curr Pharm Des 2010;16:3978–88.

31. Gao RL, Xu B, Lansky AJ, et al. A randomised comparison of a novel abluminal groove-filled biodegradable polymer sirolimus-eluting stent with a durable polymer everolimus-eluting stent: clinical and angiographic follow-up of the TARGET I trial. EuroIntervention 2013;9: 75–83.

Antiproliferative Drugs for Restenosis Prevention

Anwer Habib, MD[a], Aloke Virmani Finn, MD[b,c,*]

KEYWORDS

- Restenosis • Mammalian target of rapamycin (mTOR) inhibitors • Endothelialization • Paclitaxel

---

KEY POINTS

- Mammalian target of rapamycin (mTOR) inhibitors are the predominant anti-restenosis agent used in drug-eluting stents (DES).
- Both mTOR inhibitors and paclitaxel drugs currently approved for use in DES do not discriminate between proliferating vascular smooth muscle cells and endothelial cells and thus delay re-endothelialization and vessel healing.
- mTOR inhibitors and their analogues, while very effective in preventing neointimal hyperplasia and target lesion revascularization, can also accelerate neointimal atherosclerosis ("neoatherosclerosis"), a common cause leading to late events (ie, in-stent restenosis and thrombosis).
- Paclitaxel is an effective anti-restenosis agent comparable to mTOR inhibitors; however, the former is cytotoxic, whereas the latter is cytostatic. Both are used in DES and only paclitaxel thus far has been used on drug-coated balloons in both coronary and peripheral vasculature.
- Novel anti-restenosis agents beyond mTOR inhibitors are not being actively pursued but should be a focus of future research in order to improve vascular responses.

INTRODUCTION

Current endovascular devices in both the coronary and the peripheral vascular beds use antiproliferative agents to prevent restenosis. These antiproliferative agents mainly consist of 2 classes of agents, mammalian target of rapamycin (mTOR) inhibitors and the taxol derivative, paclitaxel. Initially, first-generation drug-eluting stents (DES) used the mTOR inhibitor, sirolimus (SRL), in 2003 (Cypher; Johnson and Johnson, New Brunswick, NJ, USA), and soon after, paclitaxel was used in 2004 (Taxus; Boston Scientific, Marlborough, MA, USA). Since then, the number of mTOR inhibitors has expanded in subsequent second- and third-generation DES to become the predominant antiproliferative agent eluted from these devices. Its use has extended into newer endovascular devices, such as the bioresorbable vascular scaffold (BVS), bioresorbable polymer DES (BP-DES), and polymer-free DES (PF-DES). Paclitaxel-eluting DES have proved to be less efficacious and more prothrombotic than limus-based DES with diminishing use in DES[1–3] in general. However, because of its particular tissue-binding characteristics, which distinguish it from limus-based drugs, it has seen resurgence in drug-coated balloons (DCB)[4] in both the coronary and the peripheral vascular beds.

Although the initial concerns with DES surround impaired endothelialization and risk of stent thrombosis, newer-generation DES with thinner struts, less polymer and drug load, and newer-generation mTOR inhibitors with specific side-chain modifications to SRL, meant to improve tissue penetration and binding, have

---

Disclosures: None.
[a] Division of Cardiology, Department of Internal Medicine, Emory University School of Medicine, 101 Woodruff Circle, Atlanta, GA 30322, USA; [b] CVPath Institute Inc, 19 Firstfield Road, Gaithersburg, MD 20878, USA; [c] Division of Cardiology, Department of Medicine, University of Maryland School of Medicine, Baltimore, MD, USA
* Corresponding author. CVPath Institute Inc, 19 Firstfield Road, Gaithersburg, MD 20878.
E-mail address: afinn@cvpath.org

Intervent Cardiol Clin 5 (2016) 321–329
http://dx.doi.org/10.1016/j.iccl.2016.02.002

reduced this risk.[2] However, current -limus agents may still contribute to overall endothelial dysfunction and the accelerated formation of atheroma (ie, "neoatherosclerosis"), leading to restenosis, late stent failure, and the need for target lesion revascularization.[2] Although current research and development of endovascular devices surround device development, there has been little research into the use and development of antiproliferative agents for local elution in vascular beds beyond -limus-based derivatives. The current -limus-based agents are discussed in addition to paclitaxel with their use in endovascular devices for restenosis prevention in addition to discussing future directions for this field.

MOLECULAR MECHANISM OF MAMMALIAN TARGET OF RAPAMYCIN INHIBITORS

SRL or rapamycin, originally discovered on Easter Island (Rapa Nui), was developed as an immunosuppressant for cancer therapeutics and as an antitransplant rejection agent in 1972.[5,6] SRL and its subsequent analogues are macrocyclic lactones, which inhibit mTOR and are part of the phosphatidylinositol kinase–related family of serine/threonine kinase. mTOR forms 2 distinct complexes named mTOR complex 1 (mTORC1) and 2 (mTORC2) by combining with different proteins with resulting complexes having distinct sensitivities to SRL (Fig. 1). Each mTOR complex integrates information from upstream signaling and controls distinct mechanisms needed for endothelial and smooth muscle cell proliferation.[7] mTORC1 is the better characterized of the mTOR complexes and integrates signaling from multiple sources, including growth factors released on arterial injury to affect process critical for endothelial coverage after injury, such as migration and proliferation.[8] SRL inhibits mTORC1 but not mTORC2 through specific binding of the FKBP12, a ubiquitous, cytosolic 12-KD FK506-binding protein and key stabilizing component of ryanodine (RyR2) intracellular calcium release channels in various cell types.[9] SRL has subnanomolar affinity to FKBP12 with 50% inhibitory concentration for the mTORC1 signaling pathway at the nanomolar range.[10] mTORC1 directly phosphorylates translational regulators, eukaryotic initial factor 4E-binding protein 1 (4EBP-1) and S6 kinase (S6K1). The regulation of proteins critical for cell proliferation and migration might in fact be the most important mechanism by which mTORC1 regulates endothelialization and neointimal hyperplasia. With vascular smooth muscle and endothelial cells, inhibition of S6K1 leads to the cytostatic effects arresting cell-cycle progression at G_0 phase, leading to inhibition of neointimal hyperplasia and endothelialization (Fig. 2). Additional inhibition of S6K1 in human endothelial cells was far more effective at inhibiting cell proliferation versus 4EBP-1.[11] Moreover, SRL effect on inhibiting endothelial proliferation could be rescued by overexpressing S6K. The relationship of SRL to TORC2 is more complex. Because short-term treatment with SRL does not inhibit mTORC2 signaling, this complex was originally thought to be SRL insensitive. However, the situation was made more complex by the observation that long-term treatment with SRL inhibits mTORC2 signaling in some cell types, including endothelial cells.[12] Less is understood about the mTORC2 complex, including its upstream effectors. It does respond to growth factors, including insulin, through poorly understood mechanisms. mTORC2 controls several kinases including Akt

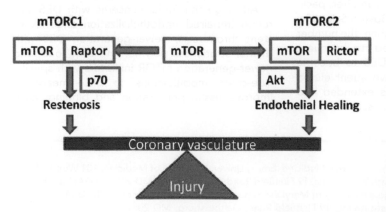

Fig. 1. The role of mTOR in vascular endothelial healing after arterial injury. mTORC1, consisting of mTOR and Raptor, phosphorylates p70, which is vital for cellular proliferation and migration of both endothelial and smooth muscle. Its inhibition leads to the prevention of restenosis after injury. However, mTORC2 positively regulates Akt activity, whose function includes endothelial survival processes such as VE-cadherins formation, which is important in endothelial barrier function and therefore healing. Current mTOR inhibitors affect both complexes in endothelial cells impairing healing after injury. Raptor, regulatory-associated protein of mTOR; Rictor, rapamycin-insensitive companion of mTOR-removed.

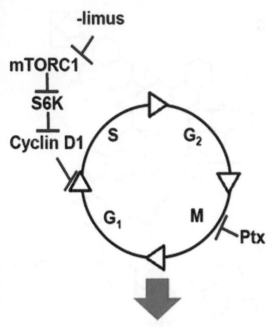

Fig. 2. Role of mTOR and Paclitaxel (Ptx) in the vasculature. Effect of -limus-based agents on the vascular cell cycle (G_1, gap phase 1; G_2, gap phase 2; M, mitosis; S, synthesis). -limus inhibits mTOR complex 1 (mTORC1) downstream effectors (S6K and Cyclin D1), arresting at G_0 to prevent S/G_1 transition. Ptx inhibits mitosis (M).

and serum and glucocorticoid-induced protein kinase 1. Inhibition of mTORC2 also likely affects endothelial recovery after DES placement by impacting endothelial survival through the

downstream effects on Akt. Akt is involved in promoting the expression of cell barrier proteins, such as vascular endothelial (VE) cadherins, important in endothelial barrier function. However, increasing evidence suggests that -limus agent's effect on barrier function may be unrelated to its effects on mTOR (**Fig. 3**).[13,14]

MAMMALIAN TARGET OF RAPAMYCIN INHIBITORS: SIROLIMUS AND ITS ANALOGUES

The use of newer, lipophilic -limus-based mTOR inhibitors (ie, everolimus, zotarolimus, umirolimus ["biolimus A9"]) have also allowed lower drug concentrations, lessening drug toxicity when compared with the prototype, SRL. Although both SRL and everolimus have been used systemically and locally,[15] newer analogues such as zotarolimus and umirolimus have been specifically developed for local elution from vascular stents. The development of locally eluted SRL analogues has been initiated by the modification of the C40 or C42 moiety on the macrocyclic ring of the SRL backbone with a lipophilic group (see **Fig. 3**). In preclinical studies, zotarolimus with a tetrazole modification to C42 had the highest lipophilicity compared with SRL and paclitaxel (**Fig. 4**),[16] allowing for rapid vascular wall uptake and pharmacokinetic titration. In in vitro modeling of both endothelial proliferation and migration, SRL appeared to have more antiproliferative and antimigratory effects on endothelial

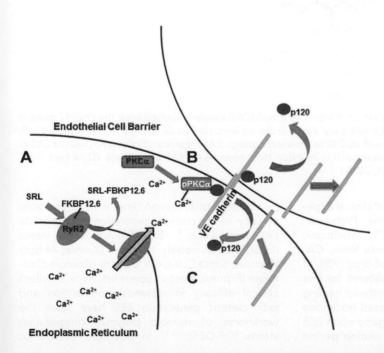

Fig. 3. Off "target" effects of SRL: impairment endothelial barrier function. (A) SRL displaces FKBP12 from RyR2 calcium release channel (blue oval) in vascular endothelial cells, resulting in increased intracellular release of free Ca^{2+} from the endoplasmic reticulum. (B) PKCα is activated and destabilized the p120-VE cadherin interaction. (C) p120 and eventually VE cadherin move from the membrane to the intracellular space leading to impaired endothelial barrier function.

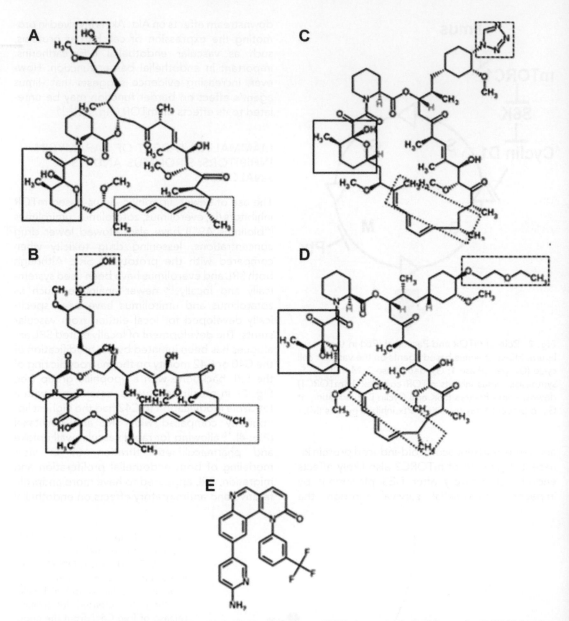

Fig. 4. SRL and its analogues. (A) SRL with its Carbon 40 group (C40) shown in dashed lines; the FKBP12 binding site shown in solid lines, and its mTOR binding site shown in dotted lines. (B) Everolimus with its C40 replaced with a hydroxyethyl group. (C) Zotarolimus with its C42 as a tetrazole group. (D) Umirolimus (Biolimus A9) with its C40 as a 2-ethoxyethyl group. (E) Torin 2, nonlimus mTOR inhibitor. Note absence of FKBP binding site. (Data from www.chemspider.com. Accessed January 24, 2016.)

cells versus everolimus.[17] The initial clinical experience with zotarolimus with the Endeavor-Zotarolimus Eluting Stent (ZES; Medtronic Cardiac and Vascular Group, Santa Rosa, CA, USA) allowed for a rapid elution of drug (90% of drug eluted by 10 days), which allowed for less vascular exposure and better endothelial healing at the potential expense of increased restenosis and late stent failure.[18] The next generation ZES (Resolute-ZES) opted for longer elution period

(~180 days total elution time) with comparable efficacy to its current generation counterparts (ie, everolimus).[6] Everolimus-eluting stents (EES), in either cobalt chromium (Xience; Abbott Vascular, Santa Clara, CA, USA) or platinum chromium (Promus; Boston Scientific), have excellent clinical efficacy in restenosis prevention and with current generation ZES have been the workhorse of durable polymer drug-eluting stents (DP-DES).[2,3,17] In addition, everolimus and biolimus A9 have been used in bioresorbable polymer DES (Synergy, Boston Scientific; BP-BES, BioMatrix),[19] polymer-free DES (PF-BES, Bio-Freedom),[20] and BVS[21] with excellent clinical efficacy in regards to restenosis prevention.[22]

Everolimus, developed in 2009 and with a C40 ethyl modification of SRL backbone, has been shown to have a more favorable vascular response in a preclinical diabetic animal model after DES implantation, suggesting it may have a role in promoting endothelial integrity, and current clinical data suggest that it may be the preferred DES in diabetic patients.[17,23,24] Despite advances in DES technology and the improved delivery and pharmacokinetics of current generation -limus-eluting stents, overall in-stent restenosis/target lesion revascularization rate at 1 year is approximately 10% without a clear advantage between current generation DP-DES in network meta-analysis between the different -limus-eluting stents.[22] In addition, multiple noninferiority studies have established the efficacy and safety of BP-DES and BVS with some valid concerns over safety (ie, stent thrombosis) surrounding first-generation BVS.[25] Although etiologic factors behind restenosis include procedural considerations surrounding stent delivery (ie, incomplete stent expansion with uneven drug delivery), resistant neointimal hyperplasia[26] (resistant to current -limus agents), and negative vessel remodeling,[27] there is a growing body of evidence that points toward the eluted -limus-based agents as contributors to late events through a common pathologic pathway involving the acceleration of atheroma formation in the neointima that overlie implanted DES (ie, "neoatherosclerosis").

NEOATHEROSCLEROSIS

Improvements in current generation DES may have largely reduced restenosis while mitigating poor endothelial coverage compared with first-generation DES, which has reduced in-stent thrombosis down to rates of 1% per year.[28] However, -limus-based DES may create what appears to be an intact endothelium that may display poor endothelial barrier function acting as a substrate for neointimal atherosclerosis known as "neoatherosclerosis" (see Figs. 2 and 3). Neoatherosclerosis is the development of foamy macrophages within the neointima, which overlie the deployed stent and is accelerated in DES compared with bare-metal stents (BMS).[29] In the authors' autopsy study of DES and BMS implants, the median stent duration with neoatherosclerosis was shorter in DES than BMS (DES; 420 [361–683], BMS; 2160 [1800–2880] days, P<.001). The

contribution of neoatherosclerosis to late thrombotic events due to neointimal plaque rupture continues to be a subject of debate. The use of -limus-based DES may contribute to poor endothelial barrier function, leading to neoatherosclerosis, which is increasingly seen as a common substrate that underlies late stent failure, leading to in-stent restenosis and potentially thrombosis via plaque rupture of the neoatheroma.[14] Previously post-mortem studies in patients with late stent failure/stent-related deaths have demonstrated both (1) poor endothelial coverage and (2) neointimal atherosclerosis ("neoatherosclerosis") as common substrates of late stent failure. Key features of neoatherosclerosis include foamy macrophages, thin cap fibroatheroma, and lipid infiltration or plaque rupture. Accelerated neoatherosclerosis is seen with first-generation DES placement (mean ~420 days) compared with BMS (mean ~2160 days) and may play a role in the greater observed incidence of late stent and very late stent thrombosis.[30] The authors previously reported in an autopsy series of first- and second-generation DES that the incidence of neoatherosclerosis was approximately 30% in both first- and second-generation (ie, EES) DES.[2]

Recently, the authors demonstrated a mechanism by which mTOR inhibition inhibits endothelial barrier formation. They showed that SRL-FKBP12 interaction impairs barrier formation by increasing intracellular calcium via destabilization of RyR2 intracellular calcium release channels and subsequent activation of calcium-sensitive protein kinase C-α (PKCα), a serine/threonine kinase important in VE cadherin barrier function through its interaction with p120-catenin (p120) (see Fig. 3).[14] This study demonstrated that the impairment in barrier formation that occurs after endothelial cells are treated with mTOR inhibitors occurs because of off-target effects of the drug itself rather than as a direct consequence of mTOR inhibition. These differences are likely exacerbated by diabetes, whereby PKCα activation is also associated with accelerated atherosclerosis, suggesting that neoatherosclerosis is likely a major contributor to in-stent restenosis, especially in diabetes.[31] These data may also explain why the incidence of neoatherosclerosis is not different between first- and second-generation DES because both use mTOR inhibitors, which use similar mechanisms (ie, FKBP12) to inhibit mTOR.

PACLITAXEL

Paclitaxel isolated from the Pacific Yew, *Taxus brevifolia*, has been used as an anti-restenosis agent in the DP-DES since 2004 (Taxus and

Ion; Boston Scientific). Paclitaxel has been highly effective as an anti-restenosis agent; however, durable-polymer paclitaxel-eluting stents overall have been shown to be inferior to -limus-based agents in major clinical trials.[22] Although there are heterogeneous data concerning diabetic patients given the concern of their resistance to -limus-based agents,[3,32] recent data suggest -limus-based DES, specifically EES, have better outcomes.[23] The molecular mechanism of paclitaxel is substantially different than -limus-based agents; it is a cytotoxic agent binding to β-tubulin and impairing microtubules disassembly and halting the cell cycle between the second growth phase (G2) and mitosis (M) (see Fig. 2). Paclitaxel, although highly effective as an anti-restenosis agent due to its cytotoxic effect, has increased fibrin formation, resulting in decreased endothelial coverage.[2] Earlier studies in animal models using different doses of paclitaxel on stents demonstrated dose-dependent increases in tissue necrosis, vascular wall hemorrhage, and delayed healing with higher doses.[33] The effectiveness of -limus-based agents may be dependent on overall cellular metabolism because mTOR signaling itself may be affected by changes in cellular nutrient status and energy levels,[34] which contribute to -limus resistance to which paclitaxel is not subject.

In addition, paclitaxel has effective vessel delivery via both DP-DES and newer DCB given its lipophilicity, especially when given in combination with excipients. The mechanism of action is related to greater and prolonged retention of the drug in tissues, likely in crystalline form, which allows release of drug up to 28 days and beyond, resulting in suppression of smooth muscle cell proliferation and persistence of fibrin with trapped paclitaxel. Although endothelial proliferation is also inhibited, due to lack of foreign body (stent), the presence the re-endothelialization is more rapid. SRL and its analogues may require constant tissue levels for a more prolonged period of time in order to be effective for restenosis prevention. Paclitaxel DCB has been effectively used for in-stent restenosis in coronary arteries previously intervened with both DES and BMS.[35] In addition, DCB has been used in peripheral vascular beds for de novo lesions (IN.PACT; Medtronic) in superficial femoral and popliteal arteries.[36] A recent

Agent	Mechanism	Systemic Use for Retenosis Prevention (Clinical Trials)	Local Elution for Restenosis Prevention	In Current Clinical Use for Restenosis Prevention
-Limus agents	mTOR inhibition	Yes (OSIRIS, ORAR III)	Yes	Yes (rarely used systemically, ie, transplant allograft vasculopathy)
Paclitaxel	Microtubule disassembly inhibition	No	Yes	Yes (local elution mainly in DCB)
Cilastazol	PDE3 inhibitor	Yes (CREST, DECLARE)	No	No
Probucol	Lipid-lowering and anti-inflammatory agent	Yes (CART-1)	Yes (tried in combination with SRL)	No
Pioglitazone	PPAR-γ agonist	Yes (POPPS)	No	No
Tranilast	Antihistamine	Yes (TREAT, PRESTO)	No	No
Prednisone	Anti-inflammatory	Yes (IMPRESS, CEREA-DES)	No	No
Colchicine	Anti-inflammatory	Yes	No	No
Torin	ATP-specific mTOR inhibitor	No	No	Investigational

Table 1
Summary anti-restenosis agents

Abbreviation: PPAR-γ, peroxisome proliferator-activated receptor-γ; PDE3, phosphodiesterase 3.
Adapted from Guerra E, Byrne RA, Kastrati A. Pharmacological inhibition of coronary restenosis: systemic and local approaches. Expert Opin Pharmacother 2014;15:2155–71.

randomized trial of paclitaxel DCB versus conventional angioplasty for symptomatic femoropopliteal disease in patients with peripheral artery disease demonstrated superior patency at 12 months with DCB (Lutonix; Bard, New Hope, MN, USA).[37]

NOVEL ANTI-RESTENOSIS AGENTS

Several systemic agents have been tried for restenosis prevention[38] (Table 1); however, locally eluted SRL, its analogues, and paclitaxel are the predominant agents in current use for restenosis prevention. The -limus-based agents' main therapeutic mechanism is through the allosteric inhibition of mTOR by FKBP12 complex, which in turn has off-target effects such as disruption of endothelial barrier function.[39] When comparing SRL with newer analogues such as everolimus, a 40-O-hydroxyethyl derivative of SRL, there is an overall decreased affinity of everolimus to FKBP12 compared with SRL.[40] These findings likely translate clinically into improved endothelial barrier function with everolimus and reduced neoatherosclerosis,[30,40,41] but definitive data supporting this concept are lacking. A role for specific mTOR inhibitors, such as ATP-competitive mTOR inhibitors (ie, torin; see Fig. 4), are potential therapeutic options for local elution in DES, which do not bind FKBP12 for mTOR inhibition.[42] These agents also have increased lipophilicity and potential platforms in DES and DCB. The use of newer more experimental agents, which selectively target vascular smooth muscle cells, may improve vascular responses to DES and enhance long-term outcomes in patients with CAD.

SUMMARY

mTOR inhibitors and paclitaxel remain predominant anti-restenosis agents with distinct mechanisms. Although mTOR inhibitors are used in various platforms in the coronaries, the use of paclitaxel is expanding in the peripheral beds and for in-stent restenosis of both bare metal and -limus-eluting stents given its increased lipophilicity and vessel wall penetration. Although there has been an expansion in endovascular device technology, there is little in the development of new pharmacologic agents for anti-restenosis.

REFERENCES

1. Daemen J, Wenaweser P, Tsuchida K, et al. Early and late coronary stent thrombosis of sirolimus-eluting and paclitaxel-eluting stents in routine clinical practice: data from a large two-institutional cohort study. Lancet 2007;369:667–78.

2. Otsuka F, Vorpahl M, Nakano M, et al. Pathology of second-generation everolimus-eluting stents versus first-generation sirolimus- and paclitaxel-eluting stents in humans. Circulation 2014;129:211–23.

3. Stone GW, Kedhi E, Kereiakes DJ, et al. Differential clinical responses to everolimus-eluting and paclitaxel-eluting coronary stents in patients with and without diabetes mellitus. Circulation 2011;124:893–900.

4. Loh JP, Waksman R. Paclitaxel drug-coated balloons: a review of current status and emerging applications in native coronary artery de novo lesions. JACC Cardiovasc Interv 2012;5:1001–12.

5. Sehgal SN, Baker H, Vezina C. Rapamycin (AY-22,989), a new antifungal antibiotic. II. Fermentation, isolation and characterization. J Antibiot 1975;28:727–32.

6. Vezina C, Kudelski A, Sehgal SN. Rapamycin (AY-22,989), a new antifungal antibiotic. I. Taxonomy of the producing streptomycete and isolation of the active principle. J Antibiot 1975;28:721–6.

7. Laplante M, Sabatini DM. Mtor signaling in growth control and disease. Cell 2012;149:274–93.

8. Finn AV, John M, Nakazawa G, et al. Differential healing after sirolimus, paclitaxel, and bare metal stent placement in combination with peroxisome proliferator-activator receptor gamma agonists: requirement for MTOR/Akt2 in PPARgamma activation. Circ Res 2009;105:1003–12.

9. Brillantes AB, Ondrias K, Scott A, et al. Stabilization of calcium release channel (ryanodine receptor) function by FK506-binding protein. Cell 1994;77:513–23.

10. Bierer BE, Mattila PS, Standaert RF, et al. Two distinct signal transmission pathways in T lymphocytes are inhibited by complexes formed between an immunophilin and either FK506 or rapamycin. Proc Natl Acad Sci U S A 1990;87:9231–5.

11. Habib A, Karmali V, Polavarapu R, et al. Metformin impairs vascular endothelial recovery after stent placement in the setting of locally eluted mammalian target of rapamycin inhibitors via S6 kinase-dependent inhibition of cell proliferation. J Am Coll Cardiol 2013;61:971–80.

12. Phung TL, Ziv K, Dabydeen D, et al. Pathological angiogenesis is induced by sustained Akt signaling and inhibited by rapamycin. Cancer Cell 2006;10:159–70.

13. Carmeliet P, Lampugnani MG, Moons L, et al. Targeted deficiency or cytosolic truncation of the ve-cadherin gene in mice impairs vegf-mediated endothelial survival and angiogenesis. Cell 1999;98:147–57.

14. Habib A, Karmali V, Polavarapu R, et al. Sirolimus-FKBP12.6 impairs endothelial barrier function

through protein kinase C-α activation and disruption of the p120-vascular endothelial cadherin interaction. Arterioscler Thromb Vasc Biol 2013;33: 2425–31.

15. Houghton PJ. Everolimus. Clin Cancer Res 2010;16: 1368–72.

16. Loh XJ, Yee BJ, Chia FS. Sustained delivery of paclitaxel using thermogelling poly(PEG/PPG/PCL urethane)s for enhanced toxicity against cancer cells. J Biomed Mater Res A 2012;100:2686–94.

17. Habib A, Karmali V, John MC, et al. Everolimus-eluting stents improve vascular response in a diabetic animal model. Circ Cardiovasc Interv 2014;7: 526–32.

18. Raber L, Juni P, Loffel L, et al. Impact of stent overlap on angiographic and long-term clinical outcome in patients undergoing drug-eluting stent implantation. J Am Coll Cardiol 2010;55:1178–88.

19. Wykrzykowska J, Serruys P, Buszman P, et al. The three year follow-up of the randomised "all-comers" trial of a biodegradable polymer biolimus-eluting stent versus permanent polymer sirolimus-eluting stent (LEADERS). EuroIntervention 2011;7:789–95.

20. Urban P, Abizaid A, Chevalier B, et al. Rationale and design of the LEADERS free trial: a randomized double-blind comparison of the BioFreedom drug-coated stent vs the Gazelle bare metal stent in patients at high bleeding risk using a short (1 month) course of dual antiplatelet therapy. Am Heart J 2013;165:704–9.

21. Haude M, Ince H, Abizaid A, et al. Safety and performance of the second-generation drug-eluting absorbable metal scaffold in patients with de-novo coronary artery lesions (BIOSOLVE-II): 6 month results of a prospective, multicentre, non-randomised, first-in-man trial. Lancet 2016; 387(10013):31–9.

22. Bangalore S, Toklu B, Amoroso N, et al. Bare metal stents, durable polymer drug eluting stents, and biodegradable polymer drug eluting stents for coronary artery disease: mixed treatment comparison meta-analysis. BMJ 2013;347:f6625.

23. Kaul U, Bangalore S, Seth A, et al. Paclitaxel-eluting versus everolimus-eluting coronary stents in diabetes. N Engl J Med 2015;373:1709–19.

24. Bangalore S, Toklu B, Feit F. Outcomes with coronary artery bypass graft surgery versus percutaneous coronary intervention for patients with diabetes mellitus: can newer generation drug-eluting stents bridge the gap? Circ Cardiovasc Interv 2014;7: 518–25.

25. Serruys PW, Chevalier B, Dudek D, et al. A bioresorbable everolimus-eluting scaffold versus a metallic everolimus-eluting stent for ischaemic heart disease caused by de-novo native coronary artery lesions (absorb ii): an interim 1-year analysis

of clinical and procedural secondary outcomes from a randomised controlled trial. Lancet 2015; 385:43–54.

26. Luo Y, Marx SO, Kiyokawa H, et al. Rapamycin resistance tied to defective regulation of p27kip1. Mol Cell Biol 1996;16:6744–51.

27. Schoenhagen P, Ziada KM, Vince DG, et al. Arterial remodeling and coronary artery disease: the concept of "dilated" versus "obstructive" coronary atherosclerosis. J Am Coll Cardiol 2001;38:297–306.

28. Waksman R, Kirtane AJ, Torguson R, et al. Correlates and outcomes of late and very late drug-eluting stent thrombosis: results from DESERT (International Drug-Eluting Stent Event Registry of Thrombosis). JACC Cardiovasc Interv 2014;7: 1093–102.

29. Nakazawa G, Vorpahl M, Finn AV, et al. One step forward and two steps back with drug-eluting-stents: from preventing restenosis to causing late thrombosis and nouveau atherosclerosis. JACC Cardiovasc Imaging 2009;2:625–8.

30. Nakazawa G, Otsuka F, Nakano M, et al. The pathology of neoatherosclerosis in human coronary implants bare-metal and drug-eluting stents. J Am Coll Cardiol 2011;57:1314–22.

31. Geraldes P, King GL. Activation of protein kinase c isoforms and its impact on diabetic complications. Circ Res 2010;106:1319–31.

32. Kastrati A, Massberg S, Ndrepepa G. Is diabetes the achilles' heel of limus-eluting stents? Circulation 2011;124:869–72.

33. Heldman AW, Cheng L, Jenkins GM, et al. Paclitaxel stent coating inhibits neointimal hyperplasia at 4 weeks in a porcine model of coronary restenosis. Circulation 2001;103:2289–95.

34. Hay N, Sonenberg N. Upstream and downstream of mtor. Genes Dev 2004;18:1926–45.

35. Loh JP, Stella PR, Sangiorgi G, et al. Paclitaxel-coated balloon for the treatment of drug-eluting stent restenosis: subanalysis results from the valentines I trial. Cardiovasc Revasc Med 2014;15: 23–8.

36. Tepe G, Laird J, Schneider P, et al. Drug-coated balloon versus standard percutaneous transluminal angioplasty for the treatment of superficial femoral and popliteal peripheral artery disease: 12-month results from the in. PACT SFA randomized trial. Circulation 2015;131:495–502.

37. Rosenfield K, Jaff MR, White CJ, et al. Trial of a paclitaxel-coated balloon for femoropopliteal artery disease. N Engl J Med 2015;373:145–53.

38. Guerra E, Byrne RA, Kastrati A. Pharmacological inhibition of coronary restenosis: systemic and local approaches. Expert Opin Pharmacother 2014;15: 2155–71.

39. Vilella-Bach M, Nuzzi P, Fang Y, et al. The FKBP12-rapamycin-binding domain is required

for FKBP12-rapamycin-associated protein kinase activity and G1 progression. J Biol Chem 1999; 274:4266–72.

40. Schuler W, Sedrani R, Cottens S, et al. SDZ RAD, a new rapamycin derivative: pharmacological properties in vitro and in vivo. Transplantation 1997;64:36–42.

41. Park SJ, Kang SJ, Virmani R, et al. In-stent neoatherosclerosis: a final common pathway of late stent failure. J Am Coll Cardiol 2012;59:2051–7.

42. Liu Q, Xu C, Kirubakaran S, et al. Characterization of Torin2, an ATP-competitive inhibitor of mTOR, ATM and ATR. Cancer Res 2013;73(8):2574–86.

Contemporary Drug-Eluting Stent Platforms
Design, Safety, and Clinical Efficacy

Ramon A. Partida, MD[a,b,c],
Robert W. Yeh, MD, MSc, MBA[c,d,e],*

KEYWORDS

- Drug-eluting stents • Percutaneous coronary intervention • Coronary stent
- Coronary artery disease • Drug-eluting stents: trends • Equipment design • Review

---

KEY POINTS

- Contemporary drug-eluting stent (DES) platforms have been developed to address high rates of restenosis seen with bare-metal stents and late adverse events seen with first-generation DES.
- Contemporary DES platforms incorporate significant advances in scaffold design, polymer compatibility, and antiproliferative drug delivery.
- DES use has become the standard of care in most clinical scenarios during percutaneous coronary intervention, including high-risk settings.

INTRODUCTION

Percutaneous coronary intervention (PCI) technology has advanced significantly since the first balloon angioplasty by Gruentzig in 1977 and eventually the first stent implantation in a patient by Sigwart and colleagues[1] 1 year later.

Initial efforts with balloon angioplasty were fraught with exceedingly high rates of restenosis, dissection, and abrupt vessel closure. These initial issues led to the development of the bare-metal stent (BMS) to scaffold vessels, leading to increased acute coronary artery luminal gain and maintenance of luminal integrity. Significant improvement in acute clinical outcomes was noted following the use of BMS, with a 20% to 30% decrease in clinical and angiographic restenosis.[2] However, vessel response to stent-mediated vascular injury leads to a significant amount of neointimal hyperplasia, vascular smooth muscle cell migration, and proliferation. This, in turn, leads to negative remodeling, restenosis, and late luminal loss, portending a high risk of need for reintervention.

The drug-eluting stent (DES) was developed to minimize the risk of in-stent restenosis. First-generation DESs have consistently been shown to decrease the risk of restenosis and need for reintervention compared with the BMS.[3] Despite proven clinical efficacy in the treatment of coronary disease, reports of adverse clinical outcomes, mostly related to stent thrombosis (ST) and late restenosis, raised concerns regarding

---

Disclosures: R.A. Partida has no relevant disclosures. R.W. Yeh has served on scientific advisory boards and received consulting fees for Abbott Vascular and Boston Scientific.

[a] Division of Cardiology, Department of Medicine, Massachusetts General Hospital, 55 Fruit Street, GRB-800 Boston, MA 02114, USA; [b] Institute for Medical Engineering and Science, Massachusetts Institute of Technology, 77 Massachusetts Avenue, E25-438, Cambridge, MA 02139, USA; [c] Harvard Medical School, 25 Shattuck Street, Boston, MA 02115, USA; [d] Department of Medicine, Smith Center for Outcomes Research in Cardiology, CardioVascular Institute, Beth Israel Medical Center, 330 Brookline Avenue, Baker 4, Boston, MA 02215, USA; [e] Harvard Clinical Research Institute, Boston, MA, USA

* Corresponding author. Smith Center for Outcomes Research in Cardiology, CardioVascular Institute, Beth Israel Medical Center, 330 Brookline Avenue, Baker 4, Boston, MA 02215.

E-mail address: ryeh@bidmc.harvard.edu

DES safety and limitation of these devices. Since the initial experience with first-generation DES, significant improvements have occurred with current DES platform technology, leading to increased safety and efficacy.[4–6] Additionally, although not the focus of this article, concurrent advances in adjunct pharmacotherapy and antiplatelet therapy have resulted in improved clinical outcomes. The sections that follow focus on the design improvements of the contemporary DES, as well as the clinical safety and efficacy of current stent platforms approved for use by the Federal Drug Administration (FDA).

COMPONENT DESIGN

DES platforms consist of 3 main components: (1) a stent metallic platform or scaffold, (2) a stent polymer coating that allows for controlled drug release, and (3) a released antiproliferative drug. **Fig. 1** shows a representative schematic the DES components.

Metallic Stent Scaffold

Current FDA-approved DES platforms are based on metallic scaffolds made of biologically inert metals with high radial strength. First-generation stents used stainless steel (SS) as the metal of choice. Recent research and development efforts have also included development of fully resorbable scaffold materials, which are currently undergoing preclinical and clinical investigation.

Although a breadth of research has focused on the advancement of polymer and antiproliferative drug components, significant improvement has also been achieved in the development of these metallic stent scaffolds. Generally, stent scaffolds are composed of 2 main components: hoops in series to provide radial strength on expansion, and connectors that join these hoops and provide longitudinal strength.[7,8] Early clinical experience, as well as insight obtained from preclinical and computational models, shed light on the role of stent geometry and strut size in deliverability; stent visibility; drug deposition; and, importantly, clinical outcomes and restenosis risk.

Initial efforts focused on optimizing stent design with existing alloys 316L-SS, such as the TAXUS Liberté stent platform (Boston Scientific, Natick, MA, USA). This allowed for reduced strut thickness of 100 to 140 μm with preserved radial strength. However, further improvement was limited by the material's moderate yield and

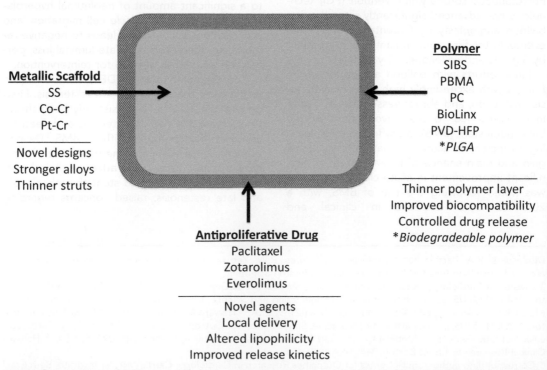

Metallic Scaffold
SS
Co-Cr
Pt-Cr
_____
Novel designs
Stronger alloys
Thinner struts

Polymer
SIBS
PBMA
PC
BioLinx
PVD-HFP
*PLGA
_____
Thinner polymer layer
Improved biocompatibility
Controlled drug release
*Biodegradeable polymer

Antiproliferative Drug
Paclitaxel
Zotarolimus
Everolimus
_____
Novel agents
Local delivery
Altered lipophilicity
Improved release kinetics

Fig. 1. Cross-section of DES strut with improved component characteristics. *, bioresorbable polymer; Co–Cr, cobalt–chromium; PBMA, poly(n-butyl methacrylate); PC, phosphorylcholine; PLGA, poly(lactic-co-glycolic acid); Pt-Cr, platinum–chromium; PVDF-HFP, copolymer of vinylidene fluoride and hexafluoropropylene; SIBS, poly(styrene-b-isobutylene-b-styrene); SS, stainless steel.

limited compression strength and visibility. Cobalt–chromium (Co–Cr) alloys used in the Vision (Abbott Vascular, Santa Clara, CA) and Driver (Medtronic, Minneapolis, MN) stent platforms have higher yield strength and modestly higher radiopacity compared with SS, and allowed for further reduction in strut thickness of 80 to 90 μm, albeit with higher elastic properties. Similarly, platinum–chromium (Pt–Cr) alloys (Promus Element and TAXUS Element stent platform) allowed for similar reduction in strut thickness and higher radiopacity given this alloy's higher yield strength.[9,10] All 3 of these alloys have been shown to be biocompatible and equivalent in in vivo preclinical models.[11] Fig. 2 depicts the stent design and major characteristic of currently available scaffold platforms.

In summary, the development of scaffolds made with these alternative metallic alloys allowed for scaffolds with smaller strut profiles with similar stent radial strength and visibility under fluoroscopy. These developments have been shown to be associated with lesser degree of arterial damage during deployment, likely reducing a stimuli for restenosis.[9,12] This holds true independent of stent geometric design.[13] In addition, scaffolds with thinner struts and decreased number of hoop connectors allow for improved device flexibility, conformability to the blood vessel, and deliverability to the target lesion; as well as theoretic improved side branch access given decreased overall scaffold profile.[7,14] Some of these design parameters seem important, not only for procedural and acute technical success, but as key drivers of drug delivery to local tissue. Stent conformability to the target vessel, stable scaffold geometric configuration, and polymer characteristics are some of the important determinants of the distribution of eluted drug.[6,15–17]

Stent Polymer Coating

Stent polymer coatings are applied to the metallic scaffold and act as drug carriers that allow for controlled local drug delivery. All except 1 of the currently FDA-approved platforms contain durable, synthetic polymer coatings that allow for predictable drug elution pharmacokinetics.

Concerns arising from reports of late ST, poor re-endothelialization, and potential hypersensitivity reactions with the use of first-generation DES platforms[18,19] led to the development of more highly biocompatible permanent polymers seen in contemporary platforms. These have been designed to induce minimal thrombogenicity at the stent surface, decrease vessel wall injury, allow for differential drug-release profiles, and lead to significant reduction in polymer layer thickness (by 40%–70%) thus decreasing the overall effective strut thickness (metal strut thickness plus polymer layer).[9] Of note, all of the currently approved DES platforms have circumferential polymer and drug elution along each strut.

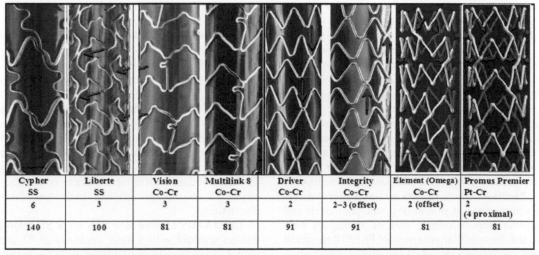

Cypher SS	Liberte SS	Vision Co-Cr	Multilink 8 Co-Cr	Driver Co-Cr	Integrity Co-Cr	Element (Omega) Co-Cr	Promus Premier Pt-Cr
6	3	3	3	2	2–3 (offset)	2 (offset)	2 (4 proximal)
140	100	81	81	91	91	81	81

Fig. 2. Stent scaffold design characteristics. Red arrows point to selected longitudinal connectors. Of note, the Promus Premier platform is identical to the Promus Element design except for the presence of 2 instead of 4 connectors in the proximal stent hoops. (Adapted from Ormiston JA, Webber B, Webster MW. Stent longitudinal integrity bench insights into a clinical problem. JACC Cardiovasc Interv 2011;4:1312; and Ormiston JA, Webber B, Ubod B, et al. Coronary stent durability and fracture: an independent bench comparison of six contemporary designs using a repetitive bend test. EuroIntervention 2015;12:1450.)

More recent research has been aimed at platforms with biodegradable polymers that resorb after drug elution. The Synergy bio-absorbable polymer (BP)-DES (Boston Scientific, Natick, MA, USA), consists of a Pt–Cr scaffold of 74 μm strut thickness, with a biodegradable poly(lactic-co-glycolic acid) (PLGA) polymer of 4 μm thickness on the abluminal surface. The polymer and drug are eluted over 4 months, after which only the metallic scaffold remains.[20] In October 2015, this platform was the first BP-DES to receive FDA approval for clinical use based on the results of the EVOLVE II trial; however, it is not yet in widespread clinical use.[20] Additional BP-DESs, such as the sirolimus-eluting Orsiro (Biotronik, Berlin, Germany), the biolimus-eluting Nobori (Terumo Corporation, Tokyo, Japan), and the novolimus-eluting DESyne BD (Elixir Medical, Sunnyvale, CA, USA), which have received the European Conformity (CE) mark but are not yet FDA approved, are outside the scope of this article.[3,21] Recent preclinical and early clinical research has focused on the use of polymer-free platforms with the use of microfabricated and nanofabricated reservoirs on the stent scaffold surface.[21]

Released Antiproliferative Drug

The eluted antiproliferative drugs are the third component of the DES platform. These are embedded in the stent polymer and are distributed into the vessel wall via diffusion in a manner dictated by local flow parameters and polymer characteristics. In this manner, the drug and polymer determine the characteristics of the vascular response and time course of vascular healing.[22]

Stent implantation induces local mechanical injury to the arterial wall and endothelium, forming a nidus for platelet activation, thrombus formation, and recruitment of monocytes, and ultimately leading to smooth muscle cell proliferation and neointimal hyperplasia.[9] Antiproliferative agents target this cellular response to reduce the rates of neointimal hyperplasia and restenosis. The main agents currently in clinical use include sirolimus analogues and paclitaxel.[3]

Paclitaxel binds to and acts as a microtubule-stabilizing agent preventing smooth muscle cell proliferation. Sirolimus and its analogues bind to the intracellular receptor of FKBP12 to inhibit the mammalian target of rapamycin, resulting in inhibition of vascular smooth muscle migration and proliferation. Additionally, it is a potent inhibitor of endothelial cell proliferation.[3,21,22] Zotarolimus is a more lipophilic analogue of sirolimus and was the first medication developed specifically for the treatment of in-stent restenosis. Everolimus is another sirolimus analogue with a shorter pharmacokinetic half-life.[3,21]

Recent preclinical research has also included the use of dual DESs that combine an antiproliferative agent with either an antithrombotic re-endothelialization promoter or a second antiproliferative agent.[21] Other novel antiproliferative agents have been developed, including novolimus (sirolimus metabolite developed for stent use), biolimus (a more hydrophilic analogue of sirolimus), and myolimus (a rapamycin derivative), which are currently being tested in early clinical trials.[9,23]

In summary, the combination of design improvements on metallic stent scaffolds, polymer technology, and antiproliferative drugs have allowed for newer generation DES platforms with improved scaffold mechanics, polymer biocompatibility, and drug-release kinetics for improved vascular endothelial healing, which have led to improved safety and clinical performance (see later discussion). Currently available DES platforms combine different scaffold designs, scaffold materials, polymers, and antiproliferative drugs, as summarized in Table 1.

COMMERCIALLY AVAILABLE, CONTEMPORARY, FIRST-GENERATION DRUG-ELUTING STENT PLATFORMS

This section provides an overview of DES platforms approved for use in the United States by the FDA, with a focus on their platform design characteristics and latest clinical safety and efficacy data.

The TAXUS Express and Cypher (Cordis, Miami Lakes, FL, USA) DES are examples of first-generation platforms that established the foundation for the development of newer-generation DES. The TAXUS paclitaxel-eluting stent (PES) consisted of a SS scaffold with a 132 μm strut plus 22 μm polymer thickness, whereas the Cypher sirolimus-eluting stent (SES) consisted of a SS scaffold of 140 μm strut thickness with a 13 μm polymer layer. These first-generation stents served as main comparators to contemporary DES in multiple clinical trials (see later discussion).

The TAXUS Liberté is a PES on a SS hybrid design scaffold with a strut thickness of 97 μm with a 16 μm thick layer of triblock polymer matrix of poly(styrene-b-isobutylene-b-styrene) and a paclitaxel concentration of 10 μg/mm2 with very slow drug-release kinetics, leading to less than 10% paclitaxel elution during the initial 28 days.[24] The TAXUS Element PES (ION stent) is

Table 1
Current drug-eluting stent platforms

Stent Name	Cypher (1st Generation)	TAXUS Express (1st Generation)	TAXUS Liberte	TAXUS Element (ION)	Endeavor	Resolute	Xience V Xpedition	Promus Element	Promus Premier	Synergy
Scaffold Alloy	SS	SS	SS	Pt–Cr	Co–Cr	Co–Cr	Co–Cr	Co–Cr	Pt–Cr	Pt–Cr
Drug (concentration, g/cm²)	Sirolimus (140)	Paclitaxel (100)	Paclitaxel (100)	Paclitaxel (100)	Zotarolimus (160)	Zotarolimus (160)	Everolimus (100)	Everolimus (100)	Everolimus (100)	Everolimus (100)
Release Kinetics	80% over 30 d	<10% over 10 d: 90% unreleased	<10% over 10 d: 90% unreleased	<10% over 10 d: 90% unreleased	95% over 14 d	80% over 60 d; 100% over 6 mo	80% over 30 d 100% over 6 mo	80% over 30 d; 100% over 6 mo	80% over 30 d; 100% over 6 mo	50% over 30 d; 80% over 2 mo
Scaffold Design	Cypher Select	Express	Liberte	Element	Driver	Driver	Multi-Link 8	Element	Promus Premier	Element
Strut Thickness (μm)	140	132	97	81	91	91	81	81	81	74
Polymer Thickness (μm)	13	22	16	15	6	6	8	8	8	4 (Abluminal)
Polymer	PEVA/PBMA	SIBS	SIBS	SIBS	PC	BioLinx	PBMA, PVDF-HFP	PBMA, PVDF-HFP	PBMA, PVDF-HFP	Bioabsorbable PLGA
Manufacturer	Cordis	Boston Scientific	Boston Scientific	Boston Scientific	Medtronic	Medtronic	Abbott Vascular	Boston Scientific	Boston Scientific	Boston Scientific
FDA Approval	2003 (no longer available)	2004 (no longer available)	2004	2011	2008	2012	2008	2008	2013	2015

Key component characteristics of current commercially available DES platforms in the United States with select first-generation DES (no longer available).

Abbreviations: HFP, hexafluoropropylene; PBMA, poly(n-butyl methacrylate); PC, phosphorylcholine; PEVA, polyethylene-co-vinyl acetate; PLGA, poly(lactic-co-glycolic acid); PVDF, poly-vinylidene fluoride; SIBS, poly(styrene-b-isobutylene-b-styrene).

Data from Refs.[3,9,14,24,25]

a next-generation system with the same polymer and drug components on a Pt–Cr open cell design scaffold of 81 µm strut thickness (Element scaffold design) that was approved by the FDA in 2011.[26]

The Endeavor (Medtronic, Minneapolis, MN, USA) platform is a zotarolimus-eluting stents (ZES) consisting of a Co–Cr open cell scaffold of 91 µm strut thickness and a 6 µm polymer layer thickness. It contains a zotarolimus concentration of 10 µg/mm stent length (or 160 g/cm^2) and a highly biocompatible hydrophilic phosphorylcholine polymer that results in very rapid drug-elution profile, with greater than 95% eluted in the initial 14 days postimplantation.[14,25]

The Resolute Integrity ZES (Medtronic, Minneapolis, MN, USA) has the same metallic scaffold and drug concentration as the Endeavor ZES (E-ZES) but contains a BioLinx polymer that is highly biocompatible and provides slower release kinetics with 85% of drug eluted over 2 months and complete elution by 6 months.[14,25]

The Xience Alpine (Xpedition or Xience Prime) (Abbott Vascular, Santa Clara, CA, USA) is a Co–Cr everolimus-eluting stent (EES) of 81 µm strut and 8 µm polymer thickness on a multilink stent open cell platform and Promus DES built on a Vision stent platform. It contains 100 g/cm^2 everolimus concentration on an acrylic and fluorinated polymer that allows for 80% of the drug to be eluted in the first 2 months postimplantation and completely by 6 months.[3,14]

The Promus Premier (Boston Scientific, Natick, MA, USA) is a Pt–Cr EES 81 µm strut thickness and 8 µm polymer thickness on an Element open cell stent platform. The polymer, drug concentration and elution characteristics are otherwise the same as the Xience Alpine Co–Cr EES.[14,25]

Table 1 shows a summary of the current commercially available stents in the United States (stent name, scaffold material, scaffold design, strut thickness, polymer, drug concentration, drug elution kinetics, FDA-approval year, and manufacturer).[3,9,14,24,25]

DEVICE-RELATED SAFETY OUTCOMES: INSIGHTS FROM MECHANICAL AND DEVICE INTEGRITY AND FAILURE
Stent Fracture
The safety of contemporary DES platforms can be evaluated from 2 distinct perspectives: (1) a device-centric model, centered on the risk of adverse events secondary to type of drug released or to mechanical device failure as determined by stent strut fracture and stent longitudinal deformation; and (2) a clinical standpoint, centered on the risk of ST and risk for target lesion revascularization (TLR).

Certain device specific characteristics have been associated with adverse clinical events. For example, certain risk factors have been recognized to increase the risk of strut fracture, which in turn has been shown to be related to higher rates of clinically evident restenosis, ST, aneurysm formation, myocardial infarction (MI), and TLR.[27–30] Some of the recognized risk factors for stent fracture include lesion complexity (eg, length, degree of calcification, vessel tortuosity, and angulation), deployment characteristic (overlapping stents, higher inflation pressure), and anatomic location (hinge points, right coronary artery, or ostial implantation).[28,30–32] Current research is ongoing in further understanding the causes, mechanisms, and underlying microenvironment stresses and strains driving this phenomenon and associated complications.[32]

Stent fracture is an uncommon complication, with a historical incidence ranging between 0.9% and 8.4%, with a 4.0% incidence on recent meta-analysis of over 5000 subjects.[31] Importantly, however, first-generation DES platforms with a SS closed-cell stent design and sirolimus elution were included and represented approximately 90% of the reported cases, while the remaining 10% were evenly distributed among all the contemporary platforms.[29] A separate registry analysis of over 9000 subjects reported a strut fracture incidence rate of 1.25% in contemporary platforms.[33] Improvement in stent design, with reduction of the number of connectors between rings from 6 S-connectors (first-generation DES, leading to decreased flexibility, stiffer stent frame) to 2 to 3 connectors in contemporary DES designs, have been largely responsible for these observations of decreased fracture despite decreasing strut thickness.

Longitudinal Deformation
Longitudinal deformation has been discussed as another potential mechanical complication of novel stent platforms, particularly given the shift toward open cell designs to allow for improved trackability while maintaining radial strength. These designs have decreased number of interconnectors between the stent rings and have been a perceived higher risk of longitudinal stent deformation or pseudofracture, which appears most commonly in the Element platform design with its distinct offset peak-to-peak interconnected ring design.[34] Although clinical outcomes with Pt–Cr EES Promus Element are similar to other second-generation DESs, bench studies suggest the Promus Element stent design has decreased longitudinal strength, making it potentially vulnerable to longitudinal shortening.[7]

Limited data are available regarding the incidence and associated clinical outcomes from longitudinal stent deformation but, in limited series, it occurs in 0.1% to 1.0% of contemporary DES platforms. It seems to be related to stent design characteristics, with a higher incidence for the offset peak-to-peak design (Promus Element platform) observed both clinically in limited, retrospective analyses[35] and in in vitro engineering longitudinal compression models.[7,36] Of note and as expected, longitudinal deformation was rarely observed with the stiffer early-generation DES platforms. Despite reports of increased risk of longitudinal deformation with novel thin-strut stents and potential association to ST[35] it seems to be a rare occurrence[37] that is mostly related to attempts to pass equipment through secondary devices during PCI.[34]

Pathologic Correlates of Stent Fracture

Pathologic and autopsy studies have shed additional light into the clinical significance of this problem. Although historical incidence was reported at 1% to 2%, autopsy studies have reported a higher incidence. However, only the most severe types of stent fractures causing gaps in stented segments were associated with adverse histologic findings on pathologic studies.[30] Contemporary Co–Cr EES platforms also seem to have decreased risk of strut fracture despite the thinner strut profiles compared with PES or SES and improved strut coverage with less evidence of inflammation, fibrin deposition, and late and very late ST (VLST). Despite these pathologic findings, fracture-related restenosis or thrombosis was comparable.[38]

Patient-Related Safety Outcomes: Insights from Clinical Experience

From a clinical perspective, and as previously discussed, first-generation DES platforms markedly decreased the risk of restenosis and have led to improved clinical outcomes. The safety of first-generation and contemporary DES platforms has centered mostly on the risk of ST. It represents a rare but potentially serious complication with a high morbidity and mortality.[39,40] First-generation DES platforms were found to have similar rates of early (0–30 days) and late (31–360 days) ST compared with the BMS.[5,41] However, safety concerns arose with reports of significantly increased, and persistent, annual risk of VLST of approximately 0.5% for up to 5 years postimplantation compared with BMS,[5,42,43] albeit with a lower restenosis and subsequent MI risk.[44]

Pathologic studies shed insight these complications because late ST and VLST seem to have distinct mechanisms between SES and PES platforms. Interestingly, SES specimens showed evidence of a hypersensitivity reaction with diffuse extensive inflammation, whereas PES specimens showed late stent malapposition with excessive fibrin deposition.[45]

Second-generation DES, with their improvements in scaffold design, polymer biocompatibility, and antiproliferative drug content, concentration, and elution kinetics, have significantly decreased this risk by addressing these failure mechanisms: pathologic studies of contemporary EES platforms have been shown to result in improved strut coverage and endothelialization, resulting in a decreased inflammatory response, less fibrin deposition, and decreased evidence of late and VLST compared with first-generation SES and PES in human autopsy analysis.[38]

A large network meta-analysis of 52,158 subjects enrolled in 51 trials with follow-up of at least 3 years, compared the long-term safety of DES to BMS up to a mean of 3.8 years, and found improved efficacy and safety profile of DES with lower rates of definite ST and target vessel revascularization (TVR), with improved efficacy of Co–Cr EES compared with earlier generation DES platforms.[46] Of note, although the EXAMINATION (A Clinical Evaluation of Everolimus Eluting Coronary Stents in the Treatment of Patients With ST-segment Elevation Myocardial Infarction) trial did not demonstrate superiority of Co–Cr EES to BMS with respect to subject-oriented endpoints in the ST-segment elevation MI (STEMI) population at 1-year follow-up, 5-year follow-up data demonstrated lower rates of these endpoints, including all-cause mortality. Importantly, TLR and ST rates were consistently lower with DES.[47,48]

In addition to meta-analyses, data from a recent large, randomized study of dual antiplatelet therapy duration has shed additional light into the safety of contemporary DES platforms. A prospective, propensity-matched analysis of subjects enrolled in the dual antiplatelet therapy (DAPT) study comparing 12 and 30 months of dual antiplatelet in 10,026 subjects (8308 with DES vs 1718 with BMS) showed a lower risk of ST with DES compared with BMS (1.7% vs 2.6%, $P = .01$).[49]

CLINICAL EFFICACY OF SPECIFIC STENT PLATFORMS

Paclitaxel-Eluting Stents

The first-generation TAXUS Express SS-PES has been found to have increasing rates of VLST compared with BMS, with reduced risk of restenosis balancing out overall clinical risk of death and MI.[42] The TAXUS Element (ION stent) represents the latest-generation Pt–Cr PES platform, which was tested against the TAXUS Express platform (SS-PES) and shown to be noninferior in the randomized PERSEUS-WH (A Prospective Evaluation in a Randomized Trial of the Safety and Efficacy of the Use of the TAXUS Element Paclitaxel-Eluting Coronary Stent System for the Treatment of De Novo Coronary Artery Lesions) clinical trial, showing no differences in angiographic target lesion failure (TLF) or clinical outcomes out to 5 years.[50] In addition, PERSEUS-SV (A Prospective Evaluation in a Non-Randomized Trial of the Safety and Efficacy of the Use of the TAXUS Element Paclitaxel-Eluting Coronary Stent System for the Treatment of De Novo Coronary Artery Lesions in Small Vessels) was a second arm of the study comparing the TAXUS Element PES against BMS with the use of historical controls from the TAXUS IV and V trials. It showed significantly lower TLR (27.2% BMS vs 14.9% Pt–Cr PES; $P = .049$) and similar low rates of ST between them (0.5%–1.0%).[50]

Newer DES platforms, however, have been found to be superior to PES platforms in multiple large clinical studies and meta-analyses, with significantly lower risks of VLST and improved event-free survival on long-term follow-up.[5,51,52] In the SPIRIT III trial (A Clinical Evaluation of the Investigational Device XIENCE V Everolimus Eluting Coronary Stent System (EECSS) in the Treatment of Subjects With de Novo Native Coronary Artery Lesions) of 1002 subjects randomized 2 to 1 to Co–Cr EES versus SS-PES, EES was found to be superior in both angiographic endpoint of in-segment late loss at 8 months, as well as composite clinical endpoint of major adverse cardiac events (MACEs) due to lower rates of MI and TLR. These results were confirmed on final 5-year follow-up.[53,54] Similarly, the SPIRIT IV trial randomized 3687 subjects to EES or PES, and showed lower rates of the primary endpoint of TLF at 1 year with EES (relative risk [RR] 0.62; CI 0.46–0.82) compared with PES.[55] Furthermore, these results are consistent with the findings from a recent meta-analyses of the final results from the SPIRIT clinical trials program showing reduced rates of all-cause mortality, MI, ischemia-drive TLR, ST, and TLF with EES.[56] Recently, the Taxus Element versus Xience Prime in a Diabetic Population (TUXEDO)-India trial randomized the latest Pt–Cr PES platform to its contemporary Co–Cr EES platform in 1830 diabetic subjects, and PES failed to show noninferiority compared with EES in the study's

primary endpoint of target vessel failure (TVF) (RR 1.89, CI 1.20–2.99, $P = .38$ for noninferiority). It showed higher rates of MI, ST, TVF, and TVL at 1-year follow-up with PES.[57]

Zotarolimus-Eluting Stents

The E-ZES platform was initially compared with its BMS scaffold base (Driver stent) and found to have lower rates of TLR in angiographic follow-up at 1 year (35.0% BMS vs 13.2% ZES, $P<.0001$) (ENDEAVOR II trial). These findings launched the ENDEAVOR clinical program, and ultimately the device's FDA approval in 2008 based on the results from the ENDEAVOR IV trial. This trial randomized subjects with de novo coronary lesions to treatment with E-ZES versus first-generation PES implantation and showed similar clinical safety and efficacy (noninferiority) in TLF despite a higher nonsignificant trend toward increased in-segment restenosis with ZES.[58] There were no differences in cardiac death, MI, TVR, or ST at 1-year follow-up. Importantly, at 5 year follow-up, there were no differences in rates of TLR (ZES 7.7% vs PES 8.6%, $P = .70$), TVF (17.2% vs 21.1%, $P = .061$); however, the rate of cardiac death or MI was lower with ZES (6.4% vs 9.1%, $P = .048$), driven by a lower rate of target vessel MI with ZES (2.6% vs 6.0%, $P = .002$). From a safety perspective, there was no difference in overall ST rates (ZES 1.3% vs PES 2%, $P = .42$); however, the rates of VLST (0.4% vs 1.8%, $P = .012$) and late MI events (1.3% vs 3.5%, $P = .008$) were significantly decreased with the use of ZES.[59]

The E-ZES platform was compared in a randomized trial to other early-generation DES with initial mixed results. E-ZES failed to meet its primary angiographic endpoint in the ENDEAVOR III trial owing to greater angiographic late loss compared with SES platforms, despite similar clinical endpoints at up to 5-year follow-up.[60] The larger ENDEAVOR IV trial eventually led to its FDA approval, whereas E-ZES was found to be noninferior to PES in a larger randomized trial with clinically oriented endpoints, although a trend toward VLST and late MI was observed in secondary analyses.[59] Subsequent trials had mixed results. The large 2333 subject SORT OUT III (Randomized Clinical Comparison of the Endeavor and the Cypher Coronary Stents in Non-selected Angina Pectoris Patients) trial in an unrestricted subject population showing higher rates of cardiac death, MI, and TVR (6% vs 3%, $P = .0002$). There were also higher rates of ST, MI, and TLR at 18 months, which leveled off and equalized owing to a higher rate of VLST with SES platforms at 3 year follow-up.[61] Further trials, however, showed higher degrees of angiographic restenosis but no increased rates of clinical events (death, MI, and ST) with E-ZES compared with SES[62] and when compared against either SES or PES.[63] In fact, a meta-analysis of these trials including 2132 subjects point to a favorable safety profile of the E-ZES compared with BMS, with very low rates of VSLT, MI, and cardiac death at 5 years; and with lower rates of TLR with ZES.[64] In the final 5-year follow-up of the E-ZES clinical trial program, E-ZES was found to have higher TLR at 1 year compared with first-generation DES; however, between 1 and 5 years, E-ZES was found to have significantly lower rates of TLR, cardiac death, MI, and ST.[65,66] Similarly, the PROTECT (Patient Related OuTcomes With Endeavor Versus Cypher Stenting Trial) trial showed a significantly lower risk of overall ST with ZES compared with SES (ZES 1.6% vs PES 2.6%, P = .003), with an improved safety profile and lower rates of VLST with E-ZES compared with SES at 4-year follow-up.[67]

The Resolute ZES, with its next-generation polymer allowing for slower zotarolimus-release kinetics, was initially evaluated in the pivotal, single-arm RESOLUTE (A Randomized Comparison of a Zotarolimus-Eluting Stent With an Everolimus-Eluting Stent for Percutaneous Coronary Intervention) trial, which showed angiographic restenosis rates of 2.1% at 9 months and 2-year TLR of 1.4% with no evidence of late ST.[68,69] This platform was subsequently evaluated against its contemporary Co–Cr EES platform (Xience V) in the RESOLUTE All-Comers trial of approximately 2300 subjects, showing similar 1-year rates of TLF (ZES 8.2% vs EES 8.3%, noninferiority P = <0.001), TLR (3.4% vs 3.9% P = .50), and ST (0.7% vs 1.6%, P = .05).[70] At 5-year follow-up, the rates of TLF, TLR, cardiac death, and MI were similar, as were rates of ST (2.8% vs 1.8%, P = .12).[71]

Most recently, the TWENTE (The Real-World Endeavor Resolute Versus XIENCE V Drug-Eluting Stent Study in Twente) trial randomized almost 1400 subjects from an unselected population with complex lesions (excluding high-risk lesions; eg, STEMI) to Resolute ZES and Xience V Co–Cr EES and showed similar rates of TVF (ZES 8.2% vs EES 8.1%, p noninferiority = 0.001), with similarly low ST rates (ZES 0.9% vs EES 1.2%, P = .59).[72]

In summary, these results and 2 recent studies comparing the Resolute ZES to newest generation Pt–Cr EES (see later discussion), show the Resolute ZES platform seems to have similar clinical efficacy and safety compared with contemporary EES platforms.

Everolimus-Eluting Stents

EES has been shown to be superior to BMS in the pivotal SPIRIT First trial, which compared Xience V Co–Cr EES with its identical Co–Cr BMS platform (Vision BMS), and showed markedly reduced rates of angiographic restenosis at 6 and 12 months.[73] It has also been shown to have a lower risk of ST compared with BMS in large meta-analyses.[74,75]

Compared with first-generation PES, the Co–Cr EES has consistently been shown to improve efficacy and safety. The pivotal SPIRIT III and SPIRIT IV trials compared the Co–Cr EES to PES and both showed decreased TLF (composite of cardiac death, MI, or TLR) at 1 year (3.9% vs 6.6%, P = .0008), with lower rates of ST (0.3% vs 1.1%, P = .003). Importantly, at 3 years, there seemed to be a decreased risk of mortality in the EES treatment arm, a finding that was confirmed at final 5-year follow-up with lower all-cause mortality (5.9% vs 10.1%, P = .02) and MACE (13.2% vs 20.7%, P = .007) with EES, despite lower but nonsignificant differences in ST, TLR, and MI.[54,55] This finding, however, has not been consistently reproduced. Another large trial (COMPARE [A Randomized Controlled Trial of Everolimus-eluting Stents and Paclitaxel-eluting Stents for Coronary Revascularization in Daily Practice]) showed improved efficacy and safety of EES compared with PES, driven instead by decreased rates of MI, TVR, and ST, without significant differences in mortality at 5-year follow-up. In this study, the rates of ST, MI, and TVR seemed to separate during the first 3 years, and then continued parallel thereafter.[76]

Randomized trials comparing Co–Cr EES with SES on the other hand, have not shown significant differences in clinical efficacy outcomes between the 2 platforms, with similar rates of TLR, MI, and death.[77–79] Differences have been observed, however, with lower rates of definite ST in EES compared with SES (0.2% vs 1.4%; HR 0.15, 95% CI 0.04–0.50) at 3-year follow-up in the SORT OUT IV trial of 2774 unselected subjects randomized to EES versus SES. As expected, this difference was driven mostly by a significant reduction in VLST with EES (0.1% vs 0.8%, HR 0.09, 95% CI 0.01–0.70).[80]

A large meta-analysis pooling more than 17,101 subjects from randomized control trials of EES versus PES or SES showed decreased rates of ST (RR 0.55, 95% CI 0.38–0.78), TVR (RR 0.77, 95% CI 0.64–0.92), and MI (RR 0.78, 95% CI 0.64–0.96) at a mean follow-up of almost 2 years.[81]

In summary, Co–Cr EES seems to have improved efficacy and safety compared with

Table 2
Key selected trials of contemporary drug-eluting stents

Trial Name	Type of Study	Stents	Number of Subjects	Longest Follow-up (Years)	Primary Outcome	Key Exclusions	Key Results
SPIRIT III[55]	Multicenter, superiority RCT	PES vs Co–Cr EES (Xience)	1002	5	In-segment late loss at 9 mo	NSTEMI, STEMI	EES superior to PES angiographically Reduced MACE at 1, 5 y
SPIRIT IV[54]	Multicenter, superiority RCT	PES vs Co–Cr EES (Xience)	3687	5	TLF at 1 y	NSTEMI, STEMI	Lower all-cause mortality (5.9% vs 10.1%, $P = .02$) and MACE (13.2% vs 20.7%, $P = .007$) with EES
ENDEAVOR IV[59]	Multicenter, noninferiority	E-ZES vs PES	1548	—	TVF at 9 mo	NSTEMI, STEMI	E-ZES noninferior to PES Trend for increased VLST and late MI in secondary analyses
PROTECT[67]	—	E-ZES vs SES	8709	4	—	None	Lower risk of VLST and overall ST
RESOLUTE All-Comers[71]	Multicenter, noninferiority	Resolute ZES vs Co–Cr EES (Xience V)	2292	5	TLF	None	ZES noninferior to EES with similar rates of TLF, TLR, cardiac death and MI, and ST
COMPARE[76]	Single-center, superiority	Co–Cr EES vs ss-PES	1800	5	Death, MI, TVR at 1 y	None	EES with decreased rates of MI, TVR, ST without significant differences in mortality
SORT OUT IV[80]	RCT	Co–Cr EES vs SES	2774	3	CV death, MI, definite ST, TVR at 9 mo	None	EES with lower rates of definite ST (EES 0.2% vs SES 1.4%, HR: 0.15), and VLST (0.1% vs 0.8%, HR 0.09)

Trial	Design	Comparison	N		Primary endpoint		Key findings
HOST-ASSURE[85]	Noninferiority, RCT	ZES vs Pt–Cr EES	3755	1	TLF at 1 y	None	No difference in TLF, clinical outcomes or rates of LSD
DUTCH PEERS[84]	RCT, noninferiority	Resolute ZES vs Pt–Cr EES	1811	1	Combined CV death, target vessel MI and TLR at 1 y	None	ZES noninferior to Pt–Cr EES Higher rates of LSD with Pt–Cr EES than Co–Cr ZES (1.0% vs 0.0%, $P = .002$)
TWENTE[72]	RCT, single-center, noninferiority	R-ZES vs Co–Cr EES (Xience-V)	1391	1	TVF	STEMI	ZES noninferior to EES Similar rates of TVF and ST
PLATINUM[83]	Multi-center, noninferiority RCT	Co-EES vs Pt–Cr EES	1530	3	TLF at 1 y	AMI	Pt–Cr EES noninferior to Co–Cr EES
PERSEUS-WH[50]	Multicenter, noninferiority RCT	Pt–Cr PES vs SS-PES	1264	5	TLF at 1 y	AMI	Similar rates of TLF (12.9% SS-PES vs 12.1% Pt–Cr PES, $P = .66$)
PERSEUS-SV[50]	Prospective multicenter, single-arm comparison	Pt–Cr PES vs BMS	224	5	Late lumen loss at 9 mo	AMI	Lower MACE and TLF with Pt–Cr PES driven by TLR

Selected key trials of contemporary DES highlighting key findings.
Abbreviations: HR, hazard ratio; LSD, longitudinal stent deformation; NSTEMI, non-STEMI; RCT, randomized clinical trial.
Data from Refs.[50,54,55,59,67,71,72,76,80,83–85].

BMS and first-generation DES, driven by lower rates of ST and VLST. Although differences in clinical efficacy outcomes have generally not been observed in trials comparing EES to SES platforms, a large meta-analysis pooling over 17,000 subjects from studies of EES versus all non-EES platforms (PES, SES, or ZES), showed that EES was associated with significantly lower rates ST, MI, and TVR, albeit with no differences in cardiac mortality.

The Pt–Cr EES platform (Promus Element) has been shown to be noninferior to its Co–Cr EES analogue in its pivotal PLATINUM (A Prospective, Randomized, Multicenter Trial to Assess an Everolimus-Eluting Coronary Stent System (PROMUS Element) for the Treatment of up to Two De Novo Coronary Artery Lesions) trial randomizing 1530 subjects to Co–Cr EES or Pt–Cr EES at up to 3-year follow-up.[82,83]

The DUTCH PEERS (DUrable Polymer-based STent CHallenge of Promus Element Versus ReSolute Integrity in an All Comers Population) clinical trial compared the Resolute-ZES with Pt–Cr EES in a randomized, noninferiority trial enrolling 1811 subjects. It showed no significant difference in the primary combined endpoint of cardiac death, target vessel MI, and TLR at 12 months (ZES 6% vs EES 5%, noninferiority $P <0.006$), or in the rates of ST (ZES 0.7% vs 0.3% EES, $P = .34$). Interestingly, there were higher rates of longitudinal stent deformation with Pt–Cr EES (1.0%) than with Co–Cr ZES (0.0%, $P = .002$).[84]

Most recently, the Harmonizing Optimal Strategy for Treatment of Coronary Artery Stenosis-Safety and Effectiveness of Drug-Eluting Stents and Anti-Platelet Regimen (HOST-ASSURE) trial randomized 3755 subjects to Pt–Cr EES or Resolute Co–Cr ZES and showed no significant difference in TLF or clinical outcomes between the 2 groups (2.9% vs 2.9%). In contrast with prior studies, however, no differences were observed in rates of longitudinal stent deformation (Pt–Cr EES 0.2% vs Co–Cr ZES 0.0%), a concern owing to the scaffold design with thin struts and offset connectors leading to less longitudinal strength when tested in vitro (see previous discussion).[85]

Table 2 shows a selected list of randomized trials of contemporary DES platforms.

CLINICAL SAFETY AND EFFICACY IN SELECTED PATIENT POPULATIONS

The safety of contemporary DES platforms has increasingly been evaluated within specific populations of interest, including high-risk subsets such as acute MI, chronic kidney disease (CKD),

and diabetes. Importantly, some of these high-risk populations are often excluded from many of the pivotal randomized trials.

Acute Myocardial Infarction

Stent implantation during acute coronary syndromes and MI remains a common clinical scenario for PCI, yet these patients were frequently excluded from many of the pivotal trials. It is associated with poorer outcomes. Initial results from first-generation DES raised concerns given significantly higher rates (RR 2.1 after 1 year) of VLST in this setting.[86] The dynamic environment during an acute coronary syndrome can lead to later stent malapposition due to thrombus, as well as potential delayed arterial healing from drug elution next to ruptured plaques.[43,87]

Computational and preclinical models shed additional mechanistic insight into potential causes for late failure with the use of DES because a thrombus present at the time of stent implantation during an acute MI modulates arterial drug distribution[88] and causes fluctuations in drug delivery.[89] Furthermore, similar models have shown that stent design (eg, thicker struts) and deployment are major drivers of thrombogenicity and appropriate polymer use reduces such risk, even in the setting of malapposition.[17]

Despite these concerns, contemporary DES platforms have been found to be safe and effective in this clinical setting. The EXAMINATION trial randomized 1498 subjects presenting with STEMI to treatment with Co–Cr EES (Xience V) versus BMS, and showed similar rates of combined subject-oriented endpoints of MI, all-cause death and revascularization, although rates of TLR were lower (EES 2.1% vs 5.0%, $P = .003$), as were rates of definite ST (0.5% vs 1.9%, $P = .019$).[48] Interestingly, at 5-year follow-up, subject-oriented clinical outcomes were significantly lower in the EES group (21%) compared with the BMS group (26%), driven mainly by reduced rate of all-cause mortality (EES 9% vs BMS 12%, $P = .047$).[47] Subsequent smaller studies have shown similar efficacy of EES compared with SES, albeit with lower rates of ST with EES platforms.[90,91]

Similarly, a network meta-analysis of 22 trials and 12,435 subjects with STEMI undergoing PCI with BMS, first-generation and second-generation DES (Pt–Cr EES excluded), confirmed an increasingly favorable safety and efficacy profile for DES, particularly with respect to Co–Cr EES platforms.[92] The exception in this clinical setting seemed to be the ZES platforms, which were found to have a significantly higher rate of TVR in this, as well as other separate analyses.[92,93]

Chronic Kidney Disease

Patients with CKD make up an increasingly large percentage, with over 40% in 1 retrospective series, of subjects undergoing PCI and DES implantation. Despite this, a scarcity of evidence exists to support its use.

Results from first-generation DES have failed to show improved efficacy compared with BMS in patients with mild to moderate CKD at up to 6-year follow-up and it has been suggested that the benefit of DES versus BMS in this population is attenuated by the altered vascular milieu.[94–96] It remains unclear whether contemporary DES use is associated with lower risk of restenosis or need for repeat revascularization compared with BMS[95] because there does not seem to be a significant difference in outcomes from DES versus BMS. As expected, a trend toward worse outcomes with PCI has been observed in the CKD population compared with patients with normal renal function.[94] Reassuringly, despite this decrease in clinical efficacy over BMS, DES use in this population has been proven to be as safe based on large retrospective propensity-matched cohort studies and registry analyses.[94–97]

Diabetes Mellitus

Diabetic patients also represent a high-risk population with historically high rates of restenosis and need for repeat revascularization. In diabetics, DES platforms have been found to have a similar safety profile to BMS if dual antiplatelet therapy is used for at least 6 months.[98] Similarly, they have been consistently been shown to have significantly lower rates of restenosis compared with BMS. A mixed-treatment comparison meta-analysis of 42 trials with 22,844 subject-years of follow-up concluded that all DES platforms were as safe as BMS (including rates of VLST) and had a significant reduction in rates of TVR (RR 37%–69%) compared with BMS.[99] Given the cumulative data, DES platforms are preferred to BMS for use in diabetic patients, although the specific DES platform of choice remains unclear. The Resolute ZES was the first to be approved by the FDA specifically for use in diabetic patients in 2012.[100] In 2015, the Promus Premier Pt–Cr EES also received FDA approval for use in patients with medically treated diabetes based on the results of the PROMUS Element Plus US Post Approval Study.

SUMMARY

DESs were developed in efforts to minimize the risk of in-stent restenosis seen with BMS. The initial concerns for high risk of late adverse events seen with first-generation DESs have significantly decreased with the use of contemporary platforms, owing to advances in scaffold design, novel metallic alloys leading to thinner struts, polymer biocompatibility, and antiproliferative drug development and delivery. Several studies, including randomized controlled trials and meta-analyses, have consistently shown the efficacy and safety of contemporary DES platforms in both short-term and long-term follow-up. Given their proven efficacy and safety profile, the use of contemporary DESs has become standard in most clinical scenarios, including high-risk settings such as acute MI and diabetic population.

REFERENCES

1. Sigwart U, Puel J, Mirkovitch V, et al. Intravascular stents to prevent occlusion and restenosis after transluminal angioplasty. N Engl J Med 1987; 316:701–6.
2. Serruys PW, de Jaegere P, Kiemeneij F, et al. A comparison of balloon-expandable-stent implantation with balloon angioplasty in patients with coronary artery disease. Benestent Study Group. N Engl J Med 1994;331:489–95.
3. Stefanini GG, Holmes DR Jr. Drug-eluting coronary-artery stents. N Engl J Med 2013;368: 254–65.
4. Cassese S, Piccolo R, Galasso G, et al. Twelve-month clinical outcomes of everolimus-eluting stent as compared to paclitaxel- and sirolimus-eluting stent in patients undergoing percutaneous coronary interventions. A meta-analysis of randomized clinical trials. Int J Cardiol 2011;150:84–9.
5. Raber L, Magro M, Stefanini GG, et al. Very late coronary stent thrombosis of a newer-generation everolimus-eluting stent compared with early-generation drug-eluting stents: a prospective cohort study. Circulation 2012;125:1110–21.
6. Garg S, Bourantas C, Serruys PW. New concepts in the design of drug-eluting coronary stents. Nat Rev Cardiol 2013;10:248–60.
7. Ormiston JA, Webber B, Webster MW. Stent longitudinal integrity bench insights into a clinical problem. JACC Cardiovasc Interv 2011;4:1310–7.
8. Ormiston JA, Webber B, Ubod B, et al. Stent longitudinal strength assessed using point compression: insights from a second-generation, clinically related bench test. Circ Cardiovasc Interv 2014; 7:62–9.

9. Martin DM, Boyle FJ. Drug-eluting stents for coronary artery disease: a review. Med Eng Phys 2011;33:148–63.

10. Sun D, Zheng Y, Yin T, et al. Coronary drug-eluting stents: from design optimization to newer strategies. J Biomed Mater Res A 2014;102:1625–40.

11. Menown IB, Noad R, Garcia EJ, et al. The platinum chromium element stent platform: from alloy, to design, to clinical practice. Adv Ther 2010;27:129–41.

12. Kastrati A, Mehilli J, Dirschinger J, et al. Intracoronary stenting and angiographic results: strut thickness effect on restenosis outcome (ISAR-STEREO) trial. Circulation 2001;103:2816–21.

13. Pache J, Kastrati A, Mehilli J, et al. Intracoronary stenting and angiographic results: strut thickness effect on restenosis outcome (ISAR-STEREO-2) trial. J Am Coll Cardiol 2003;41:1283–8.

14. Gogas BD, McDaniel M, Samady H, et al. Novel drug-eluting stents for coronary revascularization. Trends Cardiovasc Med 2014;24:305–13.

15. Takebayashi H, Mintz GS, Carlier SG, et al. Nonuniform strut distribution correlates with more neointimal hyperplasia after sirolimus-eluting stent implantation. Circulation 2004;110:3430–4.

16. Kolandaivelu K, Leiden BB, Edelman ER. Predicting response to endovascular therapies: dissecting the roles of local lesion complexity, systemic comorbidity, and clinical uncertainty. J Biomech 2014;47:908–21.

17. Kolandaivelu K, Swaminathan R, Gibson WJ, et al. Stent thrombogenicity early in high-risk interventional settings is driven by stent design and deployment and protected by polymer-drug coatings. Circulation 2011;123:1400–9.

18. Joner M, Finn AV, Farb A, et al. Pathology of drug-eluting stents in humans: delayed healing and late thrombotic risk. J Am Coll Cardiol 2006;48:193–202.

19. Nebeker JR, Virmani R, Bennett CL, et al. Hypersensitivity cases associated with drug-eluting coronary stents: a review of available cases from the Research on Adverse Drug Events and Reports (RADAR) project. J Am Coll Cardiol 2006;47:175–81.

20. Kereiakes DJ, Meredith IT, Windecker S, et al. Efficacy and safety of a novel bioabsorbable polymer-coated, everolimus-eluting coronary stent: the EVOLVE II Randomized Trial. Circ Cardiovasc Interv 2015;8.

21. Huang Y, Ng HC, Ng XW, et al. Drug-eluting biostable and erodible stents. J Control Release 2014;193:188–201.

22. Finn AV, Nakazawa G, Joner M, et al. Vascular responses to drug eluting stents: importance of delayed healing. Arterioscler Thromb Vasc Biol 2007;27:1500–10.

23. Iqbal J, Gunn J, Serruys PW. Coronary stents: historical development, current status and future directions. Br Med Bull 2013;106:193–211.

24. Garg S, Serruys PW. Coronary stents: current status. J Am Coll Cardiol 2010;56:S1–42.

25. Stefanini GG, Taniwaki M, Windecker S. Coronary stents: novel developments. Heart 2014;100:1051–61.

26. Allocco DJ, Jacoski MV, Huibregtse B, et al. Platinum Chromium Stent Series â The TAXUS Element (ION), PROMUS Element and OMEGA Stents. Intervent Cardiol 2011;6:134–41.

27. Chhatriwalla AK, Cam A, Unzek S, et al. Drug-eluting stent fracture and acute coronary syndrome. Cardiovasc Revasc Med 2009;10:166–71.

28. Park KW, Park JJ, Chae IH, et al. Clinical characteristics of coronary drug-eluting stent fracture: insights from a two-center des registry. J Korean Med Sci 2011;26:53–8.

29. Mamas MA, Foin N, Abunassar C, et al. Stent fracture: Insights on mechanisms, treatments, and outcomes from the food and drug administration manufacturer and user facility device experience database. Catheter Cardiovasc Interv 2014;83:E251–9.

30. Nakazawa G, Finn AV, Vorpahl M, et al. Incidence and predictors of drug-eluting stent fracture in human coronary artery a pathologic analysis. J Am Coll Cardiol 2009;54:1924–31.

31. Chakravarty T, White AJ, Buch M, et al. Meta-analysis of incidence, clinical characteristics and implications of stent fracture. Am J Cardiol 2010;106:1075–80.

32. Everett KD, Conway C, Desany GJ, et al. Structural Mechanics Predictions Relating to Clinical Coronary Stent Fracture in a 5 Year Period in FDA MAUDE Database. Ann Biomed Eng 2016;44(2):391–403.

33. Park MW, Chang K, Her SH, et al. Incidence and clinical impact of fracture of drug-eluting stents widely used in current clinical practice: comparison with initial platform of sirolimus-eluting stent. J Cardiol 2012;60:215–21.

34. Mamas MA, Williams PD. Longitudinal stent deformation: insights on mechanisms, treatments and outcomes from the Food and Drug Administration Manufacturer and User Facility Device Experience database. EuroIntervention 2012;8:196–204.

35. Williams PD, Mamas MA, Morgan KP, et al. Longitudinal stent deformation: a retrospective analysis of frequency and mechanisms. EuroIntervention 2012;8:267–74.

36. Prabhu S, Schikorr T, Mahmoud T, et al. Engineering assessment of the longitudinal compression behaviour of contemporary coronary stents. EuroIntervention 2012;8:275–81.

37. Kereiakes DJ, Popma JJ, Cannon LA, et al. Longitudinal stent deformation: quantitative coronary angiographic analysis from the PERSEUS and PLATINUM randomised controlled clinical trials. EuroIntervention 2012;8:187–95.

38. Otsuka F, Vorpahl M, Nakano M, et al. Pathology of second-generation everolimus-eluting stents versus first-generation sirolimus- and paclitaxel-eluting stents in humans. Circulation 2014;129:211–23.

39. Iakovou I, Schmidt T, Bonizzoni E, et al. Incidence, predictors, and outcome of thrombosis after successful implantation of drug-eluting stents. JAMA 2005;293:2126–30.

40. van Werkum JW, Heestermans AA, de Korte FI, et al. Long-term clinical outcome after a first angiographically confirmed coronary stent thrombosis: an analysis of 431 cases. Circulation 2009; 119:828–34.

41. Stettler C, Wandel S, Allemann S, et al. Outcomes associated with drug-eluting and bare-metal stents: a collaborative network meta-analysis. Lancet 2007;370:937–48.

42. Stone GW, Moses JW, Ellis SG, et al. Safety and efficacy of sirolimus- and paclitaxel-eluting coronary stents. N Engl J Med 2007;356:998–1008.

43. Nakazawa G, Finn AV, Joner M, et al. Delayed arterial healing and increased late stent thrombosis at culprit sites after drug-eluting stent placement for acute myocardial infarction patients: an autopsy study. Circulation 2008;118:1138–45.

44. Stone GW, Ellis SG, Colombo A, et al. Offsetting impact of thrombosis and restenosis on the occurrence of death and myocardial infarction after paclitaxel-eluting and bare metal stent implantation. Circulation 2007;115:2842–7.

45. Nakazawa G, Finn AV, Vorpahl M, et al. Coronary responses and differential mechanisms of late stent thrombosis attributed to first-generation sirolimus- and paclitaxel-eluting stents. J Am Coll Cardiol 2011;57:390–8.

46. Palmerini T, Benedetto U, Biondi-Zoccai G, et al. Long-Term Safety of Drug-Eluting and Bare-Metal Stents: Evidence From a Comprehensive Network Meta-Analysis. J Am Coll Cardiol 2015;65:2496–507.

47. Sabate M, Brugaletta S, Cequier A, et al. Clinical outcomes in patients with ST-segment elevation myocardial infarction treated with everolimus-eluting stents versus bare-metal stents (EXAMINATION): 5-year results of a randomised trial. Lancet 2016;387(10016):357–66.

48. Sabate M, Cequier A, Iniguez A, et al. Everolimus-eluting stent versus bare-metal stent in ST-segment elevation myocardial infarction (EXAMINATION): 1 year results of a randomised controlled trial. Lancet 2012;380:1482–90.

49. Kereiakes DJ, Yeh RW, Massaro JM, et al. Stent Thrombosis in Drug-Eluting or Bare-Metal Stents in Patients Receiving Dual Antiplatelet Therapy. JACC Cardiovasc Interv 2015;8:1552–62.

50. Kereiakes DJ, Cannon LA, Dauber I, et al. Long-term follow-up of the platinum chromium TAXUS element (ION) stent: The PERSEUS Workhorse and Small Vessel Trial Five-Year Results. Catheter Cardiovasc Interv 2015;86:994–1001.

51. Applegate RJ, Yaqub M, Hermiller JB, et al. Long-term (three-year) safety and efficacy of everolimus-eluting stents compared to paclitaxel-eluting stents (from the SPIRIT III Trial). Am J Cardiol 2011;107:833–40.

52. Stone GW, Midei M, Newman W, et al. Randomized comparison of everolimus-eluting and paclitaxel-eluting stents: two-year clinical follow-up from the Clinical Evaluation of the Xience V Everolimus Eluting Coronary Stent System in the Treatment of Patients with de novo Native Coronary Artery Lesions (SPIRIT) III trial. Circulation 2009;119:680–6.

53. Stone GW, Midei M, Newman W, et al. Comparison of an everolimus-eluting stent and a paclitaxel-eluting stent in patients with coronary artery disease: a randomized trial. JAMA 2008; 299:1903–13.

54. Gada H, Kirtane AJ, Newman W, et al. 5-year results of a randomized comparison of XIENCE V everolimus-eluting and TAXUS paclitaxel-eluting stents: final results from the SPIRIT III trial (clinical evaluation of the XIENCE V everolimus eluting coronary stent system in the treatment of patients with de novo native coronary artery lesions). JACC Cardiovasc Interv 2013;6:1263–6.

55. Stone GW, Rizvi A, Newman W, et al. Everolimus-eluting versus paclitaxel-eluting stents in coronary artery disease. N Engl J Med 2010;362:1663–74.

56. Dangas GD, Serruys PW, Kereiakes DJ, et al. Meta-analysis of everolimus-eluting versus paclitaxel-eluting stents in coronary artery disease: final 3-year results of the SPIRIT clinical trials program (Clinical Evaluation of the Xience V Everolimus Eluting Coronary Stent System in the Treatment of Patients With De Novo Native Coronary Artery Lesions). JACC Cardiovasc Interv 2013; 6:914–22.

57. Kaul U, Bangalore S, Seth A, et al. Paclitaxel-Eluting versus Everolimus-Eluting Coronary Stents in Diabetes. N Engl J Med 2015;373:1709–19.

58. Leon MB, Mauri L, Popma JJ, et al. A randomized comparison of the Endeavor zotarolimus-eluting stent versus the TAXUS paclitaxel-eluting stent in de novo native coronary lesions 12-month outcomes from the ENDEAVOR IV trial. J Am Coll Cardiol 2010;55:543–54.

59. Kirtane AJ, Leon MB, Ball MW, et al. The "final" 5-year follow-up from the ENDEAVOR IV trial comparing a zotarolimus-eluting stent with a

paclitaxel-eluting stent. JACC Cardiovasc Interv 2013;6:325–33.

60. Kandzari DE, Mauri L, Popma JJ, et al. Late-term clinical outcomes with zotarolimus- and sirolimus-eluting stents. 5-year follow-up of the ENDEAVOR III (A Randomized Controlled Trial of the Medtronic Endeavor Drug [ABT-578] Eluting Coronary Stent System Versus the Cypher Sirolimus-Eluting Coronary Stent System in De Novo Native Coronary Artery Lesions). JACC Cardiovasc Interv 2011;4:543–50.

61. Maeng M, Tilsted HH, Jensen LO, et al. 3-Year clinical outcomes in the randomized SORT OUT III superiority trial comparing zotarolimus- and sirolimus-eluting coronary stents. JACC Cardiovasc Interv 2012;5:812–8.

62. Byrne RA, Kastrati A, Tiroch K, et al. 2-year clinical and angiographic outcomes from a randomized trial of polymer-free dual drug-eluting stents versus polymer-based Cypher and Endeavor [corrected] drug-eluting stents. J Am Coll Cardiol 2010;55:2536–43.

63. Park DW, Kim YH, Yun SC, et al. Comparison of zotarolimus-eluting stents with sirolimus- and paclitaxel-eluting stents for coronary revascularization: the ZEST (comparison of the efficacy and safety of zotarolimus-eluting stent with sirolimus-eluting and paclitaxel-eluting stent for coronary lesions) randomized trial. J Am Coll Cardiol 2010;56:1187–95.

64. Mauri L, Massaro JM, Jiang S, et al. Long-term clinical outcomes with zotarolimus-eluting versus bare-metal coronary stents. JACC Cardiovasc Interv 2010;3:1240–9.

65. Kandzari DE, Leon MB, Meredith I, et al. Final 5-year outcomes from the Endeavor zotarolimus-eluting stent clinical trial program: comparison of safety and efficacy with first-generation drug-eluting and bare-metal stents. JACC Cardiovasc Interv 2013;6:504–12.

66. Maeng M, Tilsted HH, Jensen LO, et al. Differential clinical outcomes after 1 year versus 5 years in a randomised comparison of zotarolimus-eluting and sirolimus-eluting coronary stents (the SORT OUT III study): a multicentre, open-label, randomised superiority trial. Lancet 2014;383:2047–56.

67. Wijns W, Steg PG, Mauri L, et al. Endeavour zotarolimus-eluting stent reduces stent thrombosis and improves clinical outcomes compared with cypher sirolimus-eluting stent: 4-year results of the PROTECT randomized trial. Eur Heart J 2014;35:2812–20.

68. Meredith IT, Worthley S, Whitbourn R, et al. Clinical and angiographic results with the next-generation resolute stent system: a prospective, multicenter, first-in-human trial. JACC Cardiovasc Interv 2009;2:977–85.

69. Meredith IT, Worthley SG, Whitbourn R, et al. Long-term clinical outcomes with the next-generation Resolute Stent System: a report of the two-year follow-up from the RESOLUTE clinical trial. EuroIntervention 2010;5:692–7.

70. Serruys PW, Silber S, Garg S, et al. Comparison of zotarolimus-eluting and everolimus-eluting coronary stents. N Engl J Med 2010;363:136–46.

71. Iqbal J, Serruys PW, Silber S, et al. Comparison of zotarolimus- and everolimus-eluting coronary stents: final 5-year report of the RESOLUTE all-comers trial. Circ Cardiovasc Interv 2015;8: e002230.

72. von Birgelen C, Basalus MW, Tandjung K, et al. A randomized controlled trial in second-generation zotarolimus-eluting Resolute stents versus everolimus-eluting Xience V stents in real-world patients: the TWENTE trial. J Am Coll Cardiol 2012;59:1350–61.

73. Tsuchida K, Piek JJ, Neumann FJ, et al. One-year results of a durable polymer everolimus-eluting stent in de novo coronary narrowings (The SPIRIT FIRST Trial). EuroIntervention 2005;1:266–72.

74. Bangalore S, Kumar S, Fusaro M, et al. Short- and long-term outcomes with drug-eluting and bare-metal coronary stents: a mixed-treatment comparison analysis of 117 762 patient-years of follow-up from randomized trials. Circulation 2012;125:2873–91.

75. Palmerini T, Biondi-Zoccai G, Della Riva D, et al. Stent thrombosis with drug-eluting and bare-metal stents: evidence from a comprehensive network meta-analysis. Lancet 2012;379:1393–402.

76. Smits PC, Vlachojannis GJ, McFadden EP, et al. Final 5-Year Follow-Up of a Randomized Controlled Trial of Everolimus- and Paclitaxel-Eluting Stents for Coronary Revascularization in Daily Practice: The COMPARE Trial (A Trial of Everolimus-Eluting Stents and Paclitaxel Stents for Coronary Revascularization in Daily Practice). JACC Cardiovasc Interv 2015;8:1157–65.

77. Kimura T, Morimoto T, Natsuaki M, et al. Comparison of everolimus-eluting and sirolimus-eluting coronary stents: 1-year outcomes from the Randomized Evaluation of Sirolimus-eluting Versus Everolimus-eluting stent Trial (RESET). Circulation 2012;126:1225–36.

78. Kaiser C, Galatius S, Erne P, et al. Drug-eluting versus bare-metal stents in large coronary arteries. N Engl J Med 2010;363:2310–9.

79. Park KW, Chae IH, Lim DS, et al. Everolimus-eluting versus sirolimus-eluting stents in patients undergoing percutaneous coronary intervention: the EXCELLENT (Efficacy of Xience/Promus Versus Cypher to Reduce Late Loss After Stenting) randomized trial. J Am Coll Cardiol 2011;58: 1844–54.

80. Jensen LO, Thayssen P, Maeng M, et al. Three-year outcomes after revascularization with everolimus- and sirolimus-eluting stents from the SORT OUT IV trial. JACC Cardiovasc Interv 2014;7:840–8.

81. Baber U, Mehran R, Sharma SK, et al. Impact of the everolimus-eluting stent on stent thrombosis: a meta-analysis of 13 randomized trials. J Am Coll Cardiol 2011;58:1569–77.

82. Stone GW, Teirstein PS, Meredith IT, et al. A prospective, randomized evaluation of a novel everolimus-eluting coronary stent: the PLATINUM (a Prospective, Randomized, Multicenter Trial to Assess an Everolimus-Eluting Coronary Stent System [PROMUS Element] for the Treatment of Up to Two de Novo Coronary Artery Lesions) trial. J Am Coll Cardiol 2011;57:1700–8.

83. Meredith IT, Teirstein PS, Bouchard A, et al. Three-year results comparing platinum-chromium PROMUS element and cobalt-chromium XIENCE V everolimus-eluting stents in de novo coronary artery narrowing (from the PLATINUM Trial). Am J Cardiol 2014;113:1117–23.

84. von Birgelen C, Sen H, Lam MK, et al. Third-generation zotarolimus-eluting and everolimus-eluting stents in all-comer patients requiring a percutaneous coronary intervention (DUTCH PEERS): a randomised, single-blind, multicentre, non-inferiority trial. Lancet 2014;383:413–23.

85. Park KW, Kang SH, Kang HJ, et al. A randomized comparison of platinum chromium-based everolimus-eluting stents versus cobalt chromium-based Zotarolimus-Eluting stents in all-comers receiving percutaneous coronary intervention: HOST-ASSURE (harmonizing optimal strategy for treatment of coronary artery stenosis-safety & effectiveness of drug-eluting stents & antiplatelet regimen), a randomized, controlled, noninferiority trial. J Am Coll Cardiol 2014;63:2805–16.

86. Kalesan B, Pilgrim T, Heinimann K, et al. Comparison of drug-eluting stents with bare metal stents in patients with ST-segment elevation myocardial infarction. Eur Heart J 2012;33:977–87.

87. Guo N, Maehara A, Mintz GS, et al. Incidence, mechanisms, predictors, and clinical impact of acute and late stent malapposition after primary intervention in patients with acute myocardial infarction: an intravascular ultrasound substudy of the Harmonizing Outcomes with Revascularization and Stents in Acute Myocardial Infarction (HORIZONS-AMI) trial. Circulation 2010;122:1077–84.

88. Hwang CW, Levin AD, Jonas M, et al. Thrombosis modulates arterial drug distribution for drug-eluting stents. Circulation 2005;111:1619–26.

89. Balakrishnan B, Dooley J, Kopia G, et al. Thrombus causes fluctuations in arterial drug delivery from intravascular stents. J Control Release 2008;131:173–80.

90. Di Lorenzo E, Sauro R, Varricchio A, et al. Randomized comparison of everolimus-eluting stents and sirolimus-eluting stents in patients with ST elevation myocardial infarction: RACES-MI trial. JACC Cardiovasc Interv 2014;7:849–56.

91. Hofma SH, Brouwer J, Velders MA, et al. Second-generation everolimus-eluting stents versus first-generation sirolimus-eluting stents in acute myocardial infarction. 1-year results of the randomized XAMI (XienceV Stent vs. Cypher Stent in Primary PCI for Acute Myocardial Infarction) trial. J Am Coll Cardiol 2012;60:381–7.

92. Palmerini T, Biondi-Zoccai G, Della Riva D, et al. Clinical outcomes with drug-eluting and bare-metal stents in patients with ST-segment elevation myocardial infarction: evidence from a comprehensive network meta-analysis. J Am Coll Cardiol 2013;62:496–504.

93. Wang L, Zang W, Xie D, et al. Drug-eluting stents for acute coronary syndrome: a meta-analysis of randomized controlled trials. PLoS One 2013;8:e72895.

94. Green SM, Selzer F, Mulukutla SR, et al. Comparison of bare-metal and drug-eluting stents in patients with chronic kidney disease (from the NHLBI Dynamic Registry). Am J Cardiol 2011;108:1658–64.

95. Kahn MR, Robbins MJ, Kim MC, et al. Management of cardiovascular disease in patients with kidney disease. Nat Rev Cardiol 2013;10:261–73.

96. Simsek C, Magro M, Boersma E, et al. Impact of renal insufficiency on safety and efficacy of drug-eluting stents compared to bare-metal stents at 6 years. Catheter Cardiovasc Interv 2012;80:18–26.

97. Tsai TT, Messenger JC, Brennan JM, et al. Safety and efficacy of drug-eluting stents in older patients with chronic kidney disease: a report from the linked CathPCI Registry-CMS claims database. J Am Coll Cardiol 2011;58:1859–69

98. Stettler C, Allemann S, Wandel S, et al. Drug eluting and bare metal stents in people with and without diabetes: collaborative network meta-analysis. BMJ 2008;337:a1331.

99. Bangalore S, Kumar S, Fusaro M, et al. Outcomes with various drug eluting or bare metal stents in patients with diabetes mellitus: mixed treatment comparison analysis of 22,844 patient years of follow-up from randomised trials. BMJ 2012;345:e5170.

100. Vardi M, Burke DA, Bangalore S, et al. Long-term efficacy and safety of Zotarolimus-eluting stent in patients with diabetes mellitus: pooled 5-year results from the ENDEAVOR III and IV trials. Catheter Cardiovasc Interv 2013;82:1031–8.

Design Principles of Bioresorbable Polymeric Scaffolds

Mary Beth Kossuth, PhD*, Laura E.L. Perkins, DVM, PhD, DACVP,
Richard J. Rapoza, PhD

KEYWORDS

- Bioresorbable vascular scaffold • Restoration • Vasomotion • Structural integrity

KEY POINTS

- Bioresorbable vascular scaffolds follow 3 performance phases: revascularization, restoration, and resorption.
- In the revascularization phase, the performance requirements are the same for bioresorbable vascular scaffolds and drug-eluting stents.
- A bioresorbable vascular scaffold is designed to disappear over time; the restoration phase is designated by the scaffold's loss of its structural integrity to allow for gradual return of vessel functions.
- In the resorption phase, the implant is resorbed in a benign fashion, leaving behind a patent and restored vessel.

INTRODUCTION

Frequently referred to in the literature as the fourth generation of percutaneous coronary intervention (PCI), bioresorbable vascular scaffolds (BRS) are promoted as having many potential advantages relative to traditional metallic drug-eluting stents (DES). By leaving nothing behind, these include the opportunity to restore the vessel to a healthy state, capable of natural vascular function; reduce complications associated with future reinterventions and surgeries; and improve patient quality of life.

The concept for a BRS combines the best features of the first 3 generations of PCI into a single device: safe and effective revascularization (balloon angioplasty, bare metal stents, DES), suppression of restenosis (DES), prevention of constrictive remodeling (bare metal stents, DES), and long-term restoration of the treated vessel to a more natural state (balloon angioplasty). The landscape of BRS has broadened considerably since the first device to be approved, Abbott Vascular's Absorb BVS, received CE Mark approval in 2011. Several companies have introduced BRS in clinical trials around the world, encompassing new materials and targeting alternative performance goals around duration of vascular support and resorption time.

In addition to the aliphatic polyester polylactide (PLA), first used in the Igaki-Tamai device and later by Abbott Vascular in its Absorb scaffold and in different forms by many others (Amaranth, Boston Scientific, Elixir, Meril, Terumo, Xinsorb, to name a few[1,2]), several other materials are being explored for use as BRS. These include bioresorbable metals such as magnesium (Biotronik) and iron (Lifetech) and other polymeric materials such as iodinated desaminotyrosine polycarbonate (Reva).[1,2] All materials considered for such devices must be hemocompatible and biocompatible. For simplicity, the illustrative examples contained herein focus on the BRS, Absorb BVS, for which the most data

The authors are employees of Abbott Vascular.
Abbott Vascular, 3200 Lakeside Drive, Santa Clara, CA 95054, USA
* Corresponding author.
E-mail address: marybeth.kossuth@av.abbott.com

Intervent Cardiol Clin 5 (2016) 349–355
http://dx.doi.org/10.1016/j.iccl.2016.02.004
2211-7458/16/$ – see front matter © 2016 Elsevier Inc. All rights reserved.

are available (see Table 2 in this article, Bio-resorbable Scaffolds: Clinical Outcomes and Considerations by Capodanno D, in this issue).

The principles of operation of a BRS follow 3 phases of functionality, which reflect the different physiologic requirements over time, namely, revascularization, restoration, and resorption.[3,4] Most BRS designs make use of the continuum of hydrolytic degradation in aliphatic polyesters such as poly(L-lactide) (PLLA), in which molecular weight, strength, and mass decrease progressively in 3 distinct stages,[5] and the time scale of each process is adjusted to serve the in vivo need. These 3 phases, illustrated conceptually in Fig. 1, are discussed in more detail in later sections.

The challenge with BRS is to provide adequate vessel support for a minimum duration while also undergoing degradation and structural dismantling in a benign fashion and retaining vessel patency. It is this tradeoff that is of current debate as more companies explore options for BRS from both a design and material perspective.

Mechanisms for Polymeric Degradation

Given that most BRS currently available or under development are based on PLA, this material will be used as an illustration of the generalized degradation process for polymeric devices. In the initial stage, water infiltrates the polymer backbone until the material is fully saturated, which, in the case of semicrystalline PLLA, may only be about 0.5 wt%.[6] Chain scission via hydrolysis follows the hydration phase, with the amorphous regions of the polymer being more susceptible to undergoing hydrolysis. This finding results in a reduction of the overall molecular weight of the polymer backbone, with long polymer chains converted into shorter segments but still entangled (ie, molecular

weight loss without mass loss). Because initially the crystalline domains are unaffected by hydrolysis, mechanical strength is maintained even during this early molecular weight loss.

For PLA, the rate of this molecular weight loss can be determined using the equation proposed by Weir and colleagues[7,8]:

$$M_n(t) = M_n(0)exp(-kt) \qquad (1)$$

where $M_n(t)$ is the number-average molecular weight at degradation time t, $M_n(0)$ is the initial number-average molecular weight, and k is the degradation rate constant. Rearranging this equation leads to:

$$\ln\left(\frac{M_n(t)}{M_n(0)}\right) = -kt \qquad (2)$$

which enables the degradation rate constant k to be estimated from a log-linear plot of normalized molecular weight versus degradation time. This model holds true as long as no mass loss has occurred.

Eventually, water penetrates into the crystalline domains, resulting in the simultaneous reduction of both the molecular weight and the mechanical strength. As the crystalline structure disappears, progressive chain scission further reduces the polymer chains into shorter fragments until, as oligomers and monomers, they are small enough to diffuse into adjacent tissue to be either metabolized or excreted from the body. This mass loss phase will always follow after strength loss, such that a polymer scaffold will always lose its mechanical function long before significant mass loss has occurred.

PRINCIPLES OF OPERATION
Revascularization

Mechanical properties and drug delivery play prominent roles in the revascularization phase,

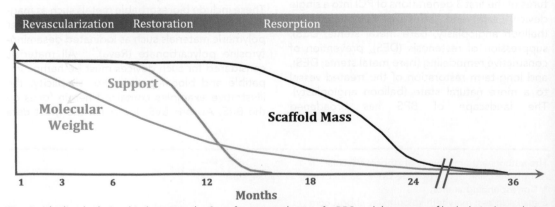

Fig. 1. Idealized relationship between the 3 performance phases of a BRS and the stages of hydrolytic degradation in an aliphatic polyester such as PLLA.

which covers the time from implantation and acute response through to the initial loss of radial support. In this phase, the BRS is intended to closely mimic the performance of a metallic DES. The BRS should be easily deliverable to the target lesion, deploy to the desired diameter to restore lumen patency, and provide sufficient radial support post-deployment to prevent acute vessel recoil and constrictive vascular remodeling. An advantage of polymeric BRS is the increased conformability and flexibility over metallic DES, allowing the vessel to maintain its native longitudinal geometry.

Another technical consideration for ensuring acute device success during revascularization is appropriate vessel sizing. This consideration becomes important at both extremes of vessel diameter. In large vessels, undersizing with incomplete strut apposition is found to be an independent predictor of worse long-term patient outcomes[9]; however, because of the inherent expansion limits of polymeric scaffolds, overexpansion can place a scaffold at risk for fracture with subsequent premature loss of radial strength or incomplete strut apposition. In very small vessels, full expansion of the scaffold to its nominal size is crucial to effect proper support of the vessel and minimize flow disturbance in an environment in which flow near the surface can represent a large portion of the vessel's total flow.

The BRS can be coated in a manner comparable to that of a DES, allowing for local drug delivery to the target lesion and controlled release over a predetermined length of time. Drug elution can be tailored to reduce the peak neointimal formation that occurs between 6 and 12 months post-implant and, thus, ensure that the artery retains patency even after mechanical support is no longer required.[10]

The idea that vessel support is not needed indefinitely but can be supplied transiently has been discussed for a long time, but one of the main points of discussion in the development of new BRS is the required duration of vessel support. Early clinical studies by Serruys and colleagues[11] and Nobuyoshi and colleagues[12] using serial angiography after balloon angioplasty found that post-intervention, the coronary lumen diameter stabilizes by 3 months. This finding suggests that a minimum of 3 months' duration of vessel support should allow for the acute revascularization provided by the scaffold to persist until such time as the vessel no longer requires it. Of the devices currently available on the market or under investigation in clinical trials, most claim to provide radial support in the

range of 3 to 6 months. Those that are not able to support the vessel for at least 3 months have had difficulty in maintaining vessel patency.[13]

During the revascularization phase of a PLLA device, the molecular weight will decrease in a predictable manner as discussed previously, whereas the radial strength stays consistently high and no mass loss occurs. Tissue coverage progresses to completion during this phase, with most apposed struts being covered by tissue at 6 months.[14,15]

Restoration

To understand the scope of the restoration phase, a brief discussion on the concepts of structural integrity within a BRS is warranted. Because by its nature a BRS is intended to disappear over time, at some point during its clinical lifecycle it will begin to lose its structural integrity. Structural integrity is considered to have 2 components: support and continuity.

Support refers to the ability of the scaffold to minimize recoil of the vessel. *Continuity* refers to the contiguity of struts throughout the scaffold. Support and continuity have different temporal performance requirements. These requirements represent the principal differences in performance relative to a DES, as all BRS are designed to develop discontinuities over their lifetime. A *discontinuity* is defined as a focal loss in continuity that does not compromise the intended function of the scaffold at that post-implantation time point. Any other loss of continuity that impairs the function of the scaffold at that post-implantation time point is characterized as a *fracture*.

In a scaffold design such as that used by Abbott Vascular's Absorb GT1 BVS (Fig. 2), consisting of a series of sinusoidal rings each connected by 3 linear links, the scaffold rings are responsible for providing vessel support, whereas the links serve to ensure uniform spacing of the rings during delivery and deployment but are not required for vessel support. The intended function of scaffold rings and links governs the post-implantation time point at which loss of continuity is acceptable. Because vessel support is required for a minimum of 3 months after implantation, the continuity of scaffold rings should be preserved for that length of time. A loss of scaffold ring continuity more than 3 months after implantation is characterized as a *discontinuity*; alternatively, should it occur earlier, it is termed a *fracture*. A discontinuity at a link after successful deployment is acceptable, as its function to preserve ring spacing during deployment is completed;

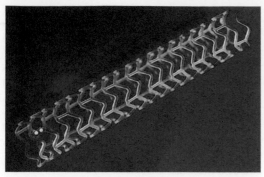

Fig. 2. Image of the Absorb GT1 BVS. (*Courtesy of* Abbott Vascular, Santa Clara, CA; with permission.)

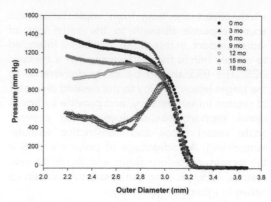

Fig. 3. Traces of pressure versus outer diameter after deployment to nominal diameter and varying periods of in vitro degradation of representative Absorb BVS 3.0×12 mm samples.

however, it is termed a *fracture* if it leads to the generation of discrete pieces before complete endothelialization. The timing constraint upon the formation of discrete pieces is dictated by the optical coherence tomography observation that 98.0% of struts were sequestered by neointima by the 6-month time point in the ABSORB Cohort B trial.[14] This observation is likely a conservative estimate of the timeframe for sufficient neointimal coverage to minimize risk of distal emboli, and with the progress to thinner-walled future BRS, this window may be reduced.

In the first 6 months, or until endothelialization is nearly complete, the requirements for a BRS closely resemble that of a DES. The restoration phase characterizes the transition from active support of the lumen to a passive implant consisting of discontinuous structural elements undergoing hydrolysis. For Absorb, based on the early clinical analysis, 6 months marks the point beyond which all types of scaffold continuity loss are acceptable.

It is during the restoration phase that there has been evidence of a return to vasomotor function, suggesting a reduction in vessel constraint.[16] This is consistent with radial strength data measured as a function of degradation time in vitro. Fig. 3 shows representative traces of pressure versus scaffold outer diameter for Absorb scaffolds tested for radial strength in the MSI RX550 Radial Force tester at in vitro degradation time points ranging from t = 0 to t = 18 months. A qualitative change in material response is noted beginning at the 12-month time point, when the scaffold transitions from ductile to brittle behavior under a circumferential compressive load. Before the 12-month time point, scaffolds are plastically deformed under a sufficiently large compressive load but still provide radial support after the yield point. Beginning at 12 months, scaffolds exhibit less

resistance to the compressive load after the yield point, suggesting a reduction in the support the scaffold can provide to the vessel. Visual observation of the units after testing show an increasing number of discontinuities after undergoing compression, which is consistent with the timescale of planned dismantling.

Adaptive or expansive remodeling is a benign and inherent feature of coronary arteries that occurs in response to physiologic stimuli, such as exercise or plaque formation (Glagov remodeling).[17] Adaptive or expansive remodeling of BRS-implanted arteries has been observed in both preclinical[18–22] and clinical studies,[15,23–25] and although the underlying mechanisms and timing between normal, healthy porcine coronary arteries and atherosclerotic coronary arteries may differ, the outcome of increased effective lumen area is the same. Timing of lumen gain is highly dependent on the scaffold, specifically its rate of degradation and loss of structural integrity, but should be considered an expected outcome of all BRS.

Resorption
After the BRS becomes structurally discontinuous, it ceases to perform any scaffolding role and may be considered functionally inert. In the resorption phase, the implant is fully resorbed in a benign fashion, leaving behind a patent and restored vessel. It is important that in the resorption phase, the degradation rate is controlled and sufficiently slow to prevent the buildup of degradation products that could incite tissue damage or inflammation. The backbone of many of the BRS under development, PLLA, breaks down into lactic acid, which is easily metabolized to carbon dioxide and water

via the Krebs cycle. Although the duration of the earlier stages of degradation may be predicted, once mass loss has occurred, there is no model for the time to total resorption. Preclinical implant experiments for Absorb have found that no measureable polymeric material remains in the scaffolded area by 3 years by gel permeation chromatography.[4]

To truly validate the benefits of a BRS, the long-term clinical result should be a completely unconstrained vessel with restored vasomotion and minimal risk of late scaffold thrombosis. At this point, the only coronary device with a significant amount of long-term clinical data is the Absorb BVS, which has shown long-term safety and efficacy and restored vasomotor function with up to 5 years of follow-up.[15,24,26]

Interesting observations related to the use of the Absorb scaffold have included an increase in mean lumen, scaffold, plaque, and vessel areas to 2 years followed by stabilization in lumen and scaffold areas between 2 and 3 years.[15] Significant regression in plaque behind the struts is coordinated with a trend toward adaptive remodeling from 2 to 3 years.[15] Absorb is currently being evaluated in several clinical trials, registries, and investigator-sponsored studies for geographically specific patient populations and in real-world applications, integrating novel primary endpoints to differentiate this technology from DES.[27–29]

SUMMARY

Table 1 summarizes the 3 performance phases, the associated performance goals, and the design considerations to achieve these goals. These 3 phases—revascularization, restoration, and resorption—are not distinct events but are a continuum of stages with the approximated durations depending on the scaffold material, its degradation rate, and its duration of maintained radial strength. Concurrent with each of these phases of the scaffold is a fourth phase of remodeling, which dependents on the vessel's response. Aside from the formation and maturation of the neointima that forms postimplant and aids in sequestering the inciting plaque, vascular remodeling begins in earnest as the scaffold declines in radial strength.[18,19] With this, the artery can undergo adaptive (expansive) remodeling to accommodate to the protective neointima and remodeling related to the regressing presence of the scaffold. This includes connective tissue infiltration into and replacement of the preexisting struts, with maturation of the replacement connective tissue to ultimately result in complete confluence with the arterial wall.[18,30,31]

One challenge remaining for BRS is identification of the proper balance of vessel support and resorption time. As more devices are investigated in clinical practice and more long-term

---

Table 1
Summary of performance characteristics in each performance phase

Performance Phase	Performance Goals	Key Design Considerations
Revascularization	• Restored patency to stenotic vessel through mechanical and potentially pharmacologic means • Re-endothelialization and neointimal sequestration of struts • Hemo- and biocompatibility	• Deliverability • Minimum acute recoil • Sufficient radial strength • Conformability • Resistant to fracture
Restoration	• Maintained lumen patency • Loss of scaffolding/radial strength through degradation and acquired structural discontinuities • Return of in-scaffold pulsatility • Return of in-scaffold vasomotility in response to physiologic (or pharmacologic) stimuli • Re-endothelialization and restoration of endothelial function • Biocompatible	• Duration of radial strength • Neointimal coverage to preclude thrombosis or distal embolization as the scaffold becomes discontinuous
Resorption	• Maintained lumen patency • Biocompatible throughout resorption	• Material biocompatibility

data are generated on devices other than the Absorb BVS, a clearer picture of the tradeoffs will be available. At the moment, clinical data from the Absorb BVS, which provide radial support for approximately 12 months before undergoing structural dismantling and achieves total resorption by approximately 3 years, has shown sustained vessel patency and restored vasomotor activity.[15] The ultimate result is a smooth lumen surface throughout the treated vessel segment with no evidence of scaffold struts as visualized with optical coherence tomography in long-term follow-up studies.[32] Further data are needed on devices that provide a shorter duration of support or faster total resorption time to understand the clinical impact.

REFERENCES

1. Tenekecioglu E, Bourantas C, Abdelghani M, et al. From drug eluting stents to bioresorbable scaffolds; to new horizons in PCI. Expert Rev Med Devices 2016;13(3):271–86.

2. Iqbal J, Onuma Y, Ormiston J, et al. Bioresorbable scaffolds: rationale, current status, challenges, and future. Eur Heart J 2014;35:765–76.

3. Oberhauser JP, Hossainy S, Rapoza RJ. Design principles and performance of bioresorbable polymeric vascular scaffolds. EuroIntervention 2009; 5(F):F15–22.

4. Onuma Y, Serruys PW. Bioresorbable Scaffold: The Advent of a New Era in Percutaneous Coronary and Peripheral Revascularization? Circulation 2011;123: 779–97.

5. Middleton JC, Tipton AJ. Synthetic biodegradable polymers as orthopedic devices. Biomaterials 2000; 21(23):2335–46.

6. Vyavahare O, Ng D, Hsu SL. Analysis of structural rearrangements of poly(lactic acid) in the presence of water. J Phys Chem B 2014;118(15):4185–93.

7. Weir NA, Buchanan FJ, Orr JF, et al. Degradation of poly-L-lactide. Part 1: In vitro and in vivo physiological temperature degradation. Proc Inst Mech Eng H 2004;218:307–19.

8. Weir NA, Buchanan FJ, Orr JF, et al. Degradation of poly-L-lactide. Part 2: Increased temperature accelerated degradation. Proc Inst Mech Eng H 2004;218:321–30.

9. Pyxaras S, Capodanno D, Gori T, et al. Impact of device sizing on outcome in patients undergoing percutaneous coronary intervention with bioresorbable scaffolds: insights from the GHOST-EU registry. Paper Presented at EuroPCR. Paris, France, 2015.

10. Virmani R, Kolodgie FD, Farb A, et al. Drug eluting stents: are human and animal studies comparable? Heart 2003;89:133–8.

11. Serruys PW, Luijten HE, Beatt KJ, et al. Incidence of restenosis after successful coronary angioplasty: a time-related phenomenon. A quantitative angiographic study in 342 consecutive patients at 1, 2, 3, and 4 months. Circulation 1988;77(2):361–71.

12. Nobuyoshi M, Kimura T, Nosaka H, et al. Restenosis after successful percutaneous transluminal coronary angioplasty: serial angiographic follow-up of 229 patients. J Am Coll Cardiol 1988; 12(3):616–23.

13. Erbel R, Di Mario C, Bartunek J, et al. Temporary scaffolding of coronary arteries with bioabsorbable magnesium stents: a prospective, non-randomised multicentre trial. Lancet 2007;369:1869–75.

14. Ormiston JA, Serruys PW, Onuma Y, et al. First serial assessment at 6 months and 2 years of the second generation of absorb everolimus-eluting bioresorbable vascular scaffold: a multi-imaging modality study. Circ Cardiovasc Interv 2012;5:620–32.

15. Serruys PW, Onuma Y, García-García HM, et al. Dynamics of vessel wall changes following the implantation of the Absorb everolimus-eluting bioresorbable vascular scaffold: a multi-imaging modality study at 6, 12, 24 and 36 months. EuroIntervention 2014;9:1271–84.

16. Gogas BD, Benham JJ, Hsu S, et al. Vasomotor function comparative assessment at 1- and 2-years following implantation of the absorb everolimuseluting bioresorbable vascular scaffold and the xience V Everolimus-eluting metallic stent in porcine coronary arteries. J Am Coll Cardiol 2016; 9(7):728–41.

17. Glagov S, Weisenberg E, Zarins CK, et al. Compensatory enlargement of human atherosclerotic coronary arteries. N Engl J Med 1987;316:1371–5.

18. Lane JP, Perkins LEL, Sheehy AJ, et al. Lumen gain and restoration of pulsatility after implantation of a bioresorbable vascular scaffold in porcine coronary arteries. JACC Cardiovasc Interv 2014;7:688–95.

19. Strandberg E, Zeltinger J, Schulz DG, et al. Late positive remodeling and late lumen gain contribute to vascular restoration by a non-drug eluting bioresorbable scaffold: a four-year intravascular ultrasound study in normal porcine coronary arteries. Circ Cardiovasc Interv 2012;5:39–46.

20. Otsuka F, Pacheco E, Perkins LEL, et al. Long-term safety of an everolimus-eluting bioresorbable vascular scaffold and the cobalt-chromium XIENCE V stent in a porcine coronary artery model. Circ Cardiovasc Interv 2014;7:330–42.

21. Virmani R. Pre-clinical bioresorbable scaffolds data. Paper Presented at EuroPCR, Paris, France. Symposium: Bioresorbable polymer scaffolds: towards routine practice in PCI. May 20, 2015.

22. Durand E, Sharkawi T, Leclerc G, et al. Head-to-head comparison of a drug-free early programmed dismantling polylactic acid bioresorbable scaffold

and a metallic stent in the porcine coronary artery: six-month angiography and optical coherence tomographic follow-up study. Circ Cardiovasc Interv 2014;7:70–9.

23. Serruys PW, Ormiston JA, Onuma Y, et al. A bioabsorbable everolimus-eluting coronary stent system (ABSORB): 2-year outcomes and results from multiple imaging methods. Lancet 2009;373: 897–910.

24. Verheye S, Ormiston JA, Stewart J, et al. A next-generation bioresorbable coronary scaffold system: from bench to first clinical evaluation: 6- and 12-month clinical and multimodality imaging results. JACC Cardiovasc Interv 2014;7:89–99.

25. Karanasos A, Simsek C, Gnanadesigan M, et al. OCT assessment of the long-term vascular healing response 5 years after everolimus-eluting bio-resorbable vascular scaffold. J Am Coll Cardiol 2014;64:2343–56.

26. Serruys PW, Ormiston J, van Guens RJ, et al. A Pol-ylactide Bioresorbable Scaffold Eluting Everolimus for Treatment of Coronary Stenosis: 5-Year Follow-Up. J Am Coll Cardiol 2016;67(7):766–76.

27. Diletti R, Serruys PW, Farooq V, et al. ABSORB II ran-domized controlled trial: a clinical evaluation to compare the safety, efficacy, and performance of the Absorb everolimus-eluting bioresorbable vascular scaffold system against the XIENCE everolimus-eluting coronary stent system in the treat-ment of subjects with ischemic heart disease caused

by de novo native coronary artery lesions: rationale and study design. Am Heart J 2012;164:654–63.

28. Kereiakes DJ, Ellis SG, Popma JJ, et al. Evaluation of a fully bioresorbable vascular scaffold in patients with coronary artery disease: design of and ratio-nale for the ABSORB III randomized trial. Am Heart J 2015;170(4):641–51.e3.

29. ClinicalTrails.gov. Absorb IV Randomized Controlled Trial (NCT02173379). 2015. Available at: https://clinicaltrials.gov/ct2/show/NCT02173379? term=NCT02173379&rank=1. Accessed February 09, 2016.

30. Onuma Y, Serruys PW, Perkins LEL, et al. Intracoro-nary optical coherence tomography and histology at 1 month and 2, 3, and 4 years after implantation of everolimus-eluting bioresorbable vascular scaf-folds in a porcine coronary artery model: an attempt to decipher the human optical coherence tomography images in the ABSORB trial. Circula-tion 2010;122:2288–300.

31. Otsuka F, Pacheco E, Perkins L, et al. Detailed morphologic characterization of the strut composi-tion following Absorb scaffold placement in a porcine coronary artery model through 48 months. J Am Coll Cardiol 2014;64:B179.

32. Karanasos A, Simsek C, Serruys P, et al. Five-year optical coherence tomography follow-up of an everolimus-eluting bioresorbable vascular scaffold: changing the paradigm of coronary stenting? Cir-culation 2012;126:e89–91.

Bioresorbable Scaffolds
Clinical Outcomes and Considerations

Davide Capodanno, MD, PhD*

KEYWORDS

- Bioresorbable scaffolds • Biodegradable stents • Scaffold • Absorb • BRS • BVS

KEY POINTS

- Second-generation drug-eluting stents (DESs), because of their permanent metallic nature, may represent a long-lasting trigger for late coronary events (ie, restenosis, thrombosis, neoatherosclerosis).
- Bioresorbable scaffolds (BRSs) eliminate this theoretic stimulus by a process of engineered resorption after the scaffold has fulfilled its purpose of stabilizing the coronary vessel for several months.
- Recently, large studies of the Absorb scaffold, with a primary or secondary focus on clinical end points, have been made available.
- Current evidence with the Absorb device supports noninferiority to everolimus-eluting stents in selected and relatively simple lesions; however, meta-analyses have recently raised concerns about a higher rate of device thrombosis compared with second-generation DESs.
- Ongoing studies with long-term follow-up will clarify the role of BRSs in daily practice. Technical ameliorations are expected to improve the outcomes of current-generation BRSs.

INTRODUCTION

Second-generation drug-eluting stents (DESs) are the current standard of choice for patients undergoing percutaneous coronary intervention (PCI) in the elective and emergent setting.[1] These devices have significantly tempered some of the traditional concerns attributed to the use of bare-metal stents and first-generation DESs. However, even second-generation DESs, because of their permanent metallic nature, represent a long-lasting trigger for late coronary events (ie, restenosis, thrombosis, neoatherosclerosis).

The principle behind the clinical development of an emerging new generation of devices for PCI, namely "bioresorbable scaffolds" (BRSs), is that of eliminating this theoretic stimulus by a process of engineered bioresorption after the scaffold has fulfilled its purpose of stabilizing the coronary vessel for several months. Although the concept of "a stent that does it job and then disappears" is intrinsically intriguing, this may come at the price of some steps back in user-friendliness and early safety compared with second-generation DESs. In fact, most BRS are made of a more fragile platform compared with metallic DESs, which limit their application and use in some PCI scenarios (ie, calcified lesions, complex bifurcations). To counteract the lower radial strength ascribable to the nature of their manufactured BRS, some companies have designed their product with thicker struts than most second-generation DESs available in the market, resulting in technical shortcomings and higher rates of early thrombosis.[2]

Disclosures: The author has received speaker's and consulting honoraria from Abbott Vascular, Stentys, Bayer, AstraZeneca, and Daiichi Sankyo.
Cardio-Thoracic-Vascular Department, Ferrarotto Hospital, University of Catania, via Citelli 6, Catania 95124, Italy
* Cardiology Department, Ferrarotto Hospital, University of Catania. Via Citelli 6, Catania 95124, Italy.
E-mail address: dcapodanno@gmail.com

Intervent Cardiol Clin 5 (2016) 357–363
http://dx.doi.org/10.1016/j.iccl.2016.02.005

However, the landscape of BRS devices is rapidly evolving and many manufacturers are now experimenting new concepts and prototypes to address the limitations of the first-generation devices. The Absorb BVS (bio-absorbable vascular scaffold [BVS], Abbott Vascular, Temecula, CA) acts as a front-runner in this challenging arena, because most of the clinical data of BRSs so far have been obtained with this particular device. For years, most of the theoretic considerations surrounding the topic of BRSs for PCI have been adapted from long-term imaging studies of the Absorb BVS version 1.0 (ABSORB Cohort A) and 1.1 (ABSORB Cohort B).[3] Although interesting and pivotal in describing the potential of BRSs at long-term (Box 1), the clinical information vehicled by these early studies has been limited. More recently, larger studies of the Absorb BVS with a primary or secondary focus on clinical end points have been made available. In parallel, several manufacturers are at the beginning of their line of clinical development of competing BRSs. This article reviews the contemporary clinical outcomes of the Absorb BVS, and provides an updated state of the art on the other players in the BRS field.

CLINICAL DEVELOPMENT OF CURRENT-GENERATION BIORESORBABLE SCAFFOLDS

Three polymeric BRS have currently obtained the CE mark for use in Europe: Absorb, DESolve (Elixir, Sunnyvale, CA), and ART (Arterial Resorbable Technologies, Noisy le Roi, France and Terumo, Tokyo, Japan). Absorb is so far the only BRS that has been approved by the US Food and Drug Administration. Other BRSs in the early stages of clinical development include the polymeric Fortitude (Amaranth Medical, Mountain View, CA), NeoVas (Lepu Medical Technology, Beijing, China), Mirage (Manli, Singapore, Singapore), MeRes (Meril Life Sciences, Gujarat, India), Xinsorb (Huaan Biotechnology, Laiwu, China), Fantom (REVA Medical, San Diego, CA), and the metallic DREAMS (Biotronik AG, Aarau, Switzerland) (Table 1). Other BRS are still in preclinical testing and have not launched an official clinical development program, such as ON-AVS (OrbusNeich Medical, Ft. Lauderdale, FL), ZMED (Zorion Medical, Zionsville, IN), Sahajanand BRS (Sahajanand Medical Technologies, Gujarat, India), Avatar BRS (S3V, Karnataka, India), Stanza BRS (480 Biomedical, Watertown, MA), Biolute (Envision Scientific, Gujarat, India), and ArterioSorb (Arterius, Bradford, United Kingdom).

Absorb

Absorb is the BRS with the most extensive clinical evaluation so far, and several randomized studies versus everolimus-eluting stents (EESs) have been published recently:

- A small investigator-driven trial named EVERBIO II concluded that second-generation metallic DESs (EESs or biolimus-eluting stents) were not superior to the Absorb BVS in terms of

---

Box 1
Predicated advantages of bioresorbable scaffolds

Superior conformability and flexibility
- Improved distribution of tissue biomechanics
- Preserved vessel geometry

Liberation of vessel from a metallic cage
- Restoration of physiologic vasomotion, adaptive shear stress, late luminal gain, and late expansive remodeling

Absence of any residual foreign material and restoration of functional endothelial coverage
- Reduced risk of late thrombosis
- Reduced need for long-term dual antiplatelet therapy

Additional technical benefits
- No "jailing" of the side branches
- No overhang at ostial lesions
- No inability to graft the stented segment
- No artifacts on computed tomography

Table 1
Summary of design, structure, and resorption time of current-generation BRS (approved or under clinical testing)

Scaffold	Company	Strut Material	Drug	Strut (μm)	Resorption (mo)	Status
Absorb GT1 BVS	Abbott Vascular	PLA	Everolimus	156	24–36	CE mark
DESolve	Elixir	PLA	Novolimus	150	24–36	CE mark
ART PBS	Terumo/ART	PLA	—	170	12–24	CE mark
Fortitude	Amaranth Medical	PLA	—	120	12–24	On clinical studies
NeoVas	Lepu Medical Technology	PLA	Sirolimus	180	NA	On clinical studies
Mirage	Manli	PLA	—	125–150	14	On clinical studies
MeRes100	Meril LifeSciences	PLA	—	100	24	On clinical studies
Xinsorb	Huaan Biotch	PLA	Sirolimus	150–160	NA	On clinical studies
Fantom	REVA Medical	DT-PC	Sirolimus	NA	NA	On clinical studies
DREAMS-2G	Biotronik	Magnesium	Sirolimus	120–150	12	On clinical studies

Abbreviations: BVS, bioresorbable vascular scaffold; DT-PC, desaminotyrosine polycarbonate; NA, not available; PBS, pure bioresorbable scaffold; PLA, Polylactide acid.

9-month angiographic late loss and clinical outcomes.[4]

- ABSORB II is an ongoing study powered to detect differences in the coprimary surrogate end points of vasomotion and lumen loss at 3 years.[5] Preliminary data have been reported that show similar 1-year composite secondary clinical outcomes of the Absorb BVS compared with EES, but this study is underpowered for detecting differences in clinical end points.[6]
- In ABSORB STEMI-TROFI II, another independent comparison of Absorb BVSs and EESs, stenting of the culprit lesions with the Absorb BVS in the setting of ST-segment elevation myocardial infarction, resulted in nearly complete arterial healing that was comparable with that of EESs at 6 months, and the rates of target lesion failure (TLF) were similarly low.[7]

A series of larger randomized studies to support local regulatory approval of the ABSORB BVS have been also completed:

- In ABSORB JAPAN, the 1-year clinical and 13-month angiographic outcomes of the

Absorb BVS were comparable with those of the EES.[8]

- In ABSORB China, the Absorb BVS was noninferior to the EES for the primary end point of in-segment late loss at 1 year, with similar rates of TLF and definite or probable device thrombosis.[9]
- ABSORB III (the regulatory trial for the United States) is so far the only trial powered for clinical end points. Compared with the EES, the Absorb BVS was within the prespecified margin for noninferiority with respect to TLF at 1 year, although the rates of subacute device thrombosis were greater.[10]

When appraising the results of these early studies, one should take into account the relative simplicity of the patient and lesion included, and with the possible exception of ABSORB III (N = 2008) the small number of patients randomized. This results in multiple end points (ie, myocardial infarction, device thrombosis) showing no nominal significant difference between Absorb BVSs and EESs as the mere reflection of a type II error (ie, false-negative findings caused by the small number of subjects randomized). Recently, a meta-analysis of the six randomized trials described previously pooled a total of 3738 patients undergoing PCI with Absorb BVSs (N = 2337) or EESs (N = 1401).[11] At a median follow-up of 12 months, there was no difference in all-cause mortality, but patients who received Absorb BVSs had a significantly higher risk of definite or probable device thrombosis (odds ratio [OR], 1.99; 95% confidence interval [CI], 1.00–3.98; P = .05), subacute device thrombosis (OR, 3.11; 95% CI, 1.24–7.82; P = .02), and a numerically higher risk of myocardial infarction (OR, 1.36; 95% CI, 0.98–1.89; P = .06) than those treated with EES. The risks of target lesion revascularization and TLF were similar between Absorb BVSs and EESs, despite the poorer angiographic performance of the former reflected by greater in-device lumen loss at mid-term. Consistently, another meta-analysis including 10,510 patients from randomized clinical trials and registries, such as the large real-world GHOST-EU,[12] reported a two-fold increased risk of myocardial infarction and definite or probable device thrombosis with BRSs compared with DESs.[13]

In summary, when simple candidates and lesions are taken into considerations, the risk of 12-month repeat revascularization with the Absorb BVSs resembles that of EESs, implying an acceptable mechanical performance in the mid-term. However, this comes at the price of higher rates of stent thrombosis (clustering mostly between 1 and 30 days after implantation) and myocardial infarction. In view of this, the net benefit of implanting Absorb BVSs is difficult to capture, because of limited follow-up information from the available trials, rarely extending beyond 1 year. Theoretically, the poorer mid-term safety profile of BRS could be offset by later benefits emerging after bioresorption (ie, lower rates of late TLF and device thrombosis) (see Box 1). This hypothesis is currently tested in the ABSORB IV trial (NCT02173379), a study of approximately 5000 subjects (~2000 primary analysis subjects of ABSORB III and ~3000 subjects of ABSORB IV) powered to test the noninferiority of the Absorb BVS to the EES.

DESolve

The DESolve BRS has been tested in the DESolve first-in-man study, where 16 patients underwent scaffold implantation.[14] Late loss was 0.19 ± 0.19 mm at 6 months, and at 12 months there was no reported scaffold thrombosis or major adverse cardiac events. DESolve Nx was a multicenter, prospective single-arm study of a subsequent generation of the device incorporating another antiproliferative drug (ie,

novolimus instead of myolimus) and enrolling 126 patients. The primary end point of late loss at 6 months was 0.20 ± 0.32 mm. At 36 months follow-up, TLF was 8.2%, including cardiac death in 3.3%, target vessel myocardial infarction in 0.8%, clinically indicated TLR in 4.1%, and no case of scaffold thrombosis (Abizaid A, Transcatheter Cardiovascular Therapeutics 2015, San Francisco).

ART

The ART BRS, which is not drug-eluting, has so far been investigated only in preclinical models and the multicenter first-in-man ARTDIVA trial. In the latter, out of 30 treated patients, three (10%) repeat revascularizations have been reported at 6 months (only one was ischemia-driven), with no cases of cardiac death or myocardial infarction (Lafont A, Transcatheter Cardiovascular Therapeutics 2015, San Francisco). The scaffold has received CE Mark clearance in Europe (where is still not currently marketed at the time of drafting this article), and the manufacturers have announced the planned development of a drug-eluting version of the scaffold.

Fortitude

After preclinical and early clinical testing of a now abandoned non-drug-eluting version, the sirolimus-eluting BRS Fortitude (150 μm) is currently being tested in the RENASCENT first-in-man study, enrolling 63 patients, whose results are pending. Preliminary results of the first 13 patients have been reported (Granada J, Transcatheter Cardiovascular Therapeutics 2015, San Francisco), showing 7.7% of target vessel failure at 9 months because of one periprocedural myocardial infarction, with no case of restenosis or thrombosis. Recently, the investigators announced plans to initiate RENASCENT II, a new first-in-man study of the second-generation Fortitude BRS, featuring a thinner-strut iteration (120 μm) of the device. Testing of an even thinner (90 μm) version of the device is planned.

NeoVas

A first-in-man study of the Neo-Vas BRS has been launched, recruiting 31 patients. The authors reported TLF at 1 year in 3.2% (Granada J, Transcatheter Cardiovascular Therapeutics 2015, San Francisco), and announced the launch of a randomized study of 560 patients comparing NeoVas with EESs. Coprimary end points for this randomized trial will be late loss at 1 year and vasomotion at 3 years.

Mirage

The Mirage BRS has been compared with the Absorb BRS in a randomized trial of 68 patients, named MIRAGE. The primary end point, in-scaffold late lumen loss at 12 months, is pending. Preliminary 6-month results have recently being reported, suggesting a comparable performance between devices in terms of in-scaffold diameter performance derived from optical coherence tomography area measurements (Santoso T, Transcatheter Cardiovascular Therapeutics 2015, San Francisco).

MeRes

The first-in-man study of the MeRes100 BRS, named MeRes-1, is going to enroll 108 patients at 16 Indian sites (Leon M, Transcatheter Cardiovascular Therapeutics 2015, San Francisco). The manufacturer has also announced the initiation of other registries (ie, MeRes Global) and two randomized clinical trials versus the Absorb BVS (MeRes100-China, and MeRes-Evolve).

Xinsorb

The first-in-man study of the Xinsorb BRS has included 30 patients. At 6 months, late lumen loss has been estimated at 0.17 ± 0.12 mm, with one case of TLF at 18 months (3.7%) attributable to a nonfatal definite thrombosis (Ge L, Transcatheter Cardiovascular Therapeutics 2015, San Francisco). The manufacturer has started a randomized study versus a biodegradable-polymer DES, and a single-arm registry of 800 patients.

Fantom

Fantom is the evolution of the former ReZolve and ReZolve-2 BRSs, formerly tested in the RESTORE and RESTORE-II studies. The FANTOM I clinical trial, which began enrolling patients with Fantom in December 2014, is being conducted to provide early clinical data. The manufacturer has recently announced the initiation of a CE clinical trial (FANTOM II) enrolling a minimum of 110 patients.

DREAMS

The DREAMS-2G BRS has been tested in the BIOSOLVE-II study, whose primary end point (late lumen loss) has been the object of a recent publication.[15] The trial was a single-arm, first-in-man investigation of a second-generation BRS developed to introduce device ameliorations, focusing on surrogate end points. The investigators reported a late loss of 0.27 ± 0.37 mm in 123 patients at 6 months, and intravascular ultrasound assessment showed preservation of the scaffold area and low mean neointimal area.

TLF occurred in 3% of patients, and no definite or probable scaffold thrombosis was observed. Importantly, DREAMS-2 represents the evolution of the former non-drug-eluting version of the scaffold (AMS-1) and the earlier drug-eluting version (DREAMS-1), evaluated respectively in the PROGRESS-AMS[16,17] and BIOSOLVE-I studies.[18] The results of BIOSOLVE-II do not support firm conclusions on the safety and efficacy of DREAMS-2 on a clinical ground, but support further testing of metal BRS as an alternative to polymeric BRS.

QUO VADIS, BIORESORBABLE SCAFFOLD?

It is difficult to anticipate the future of BRSs in the next 10 or so years. Clearly, the principle behind using BRSs for PCI is worthy of attention. Caging the coronary arteries with metallic stents has historically reduced the amount of recurrences, but the focus of the discussion is now on the role and responsibility of durable metal in the onset of long-term events. Adding to stent thrombosis, some advocate a series of other long-term disadvantages of DESs, which include loss of vasomotion ability, mechanotransduction, adaptive shear stress, late luminal gain, and expansive remodeling (Fig. 1).[3] The early studies of the Absorb BVS have underscored the potential role of BRSs in restoring these functions, but the clinical impact of such improvements remains unknown. One may advocate that recovery of vasomotion and liberation from mechanical distortion may have beneficial effects on the rates of post-PCI angina. Indeed, angina seriously affects the quality of life, and remains an unsolved issue in a proportion of patients who have undergone PCI. The ABSORB II trial suggests that BRSs may reduce angina compared with EESs, but this finding was based on site-reported assessment by study staff potentially aware of treatment allocation. Importantly, angina reduction benefits have not been confirmed in ABSORB III. Indeed, angina is a challenging end point in clinical trial design, because of its subjective nature in patient's reporting and physician's assessment. ABSORB IV will include 3000 patients for a powered comparison of angina rates at 1 year, featuring a sophisticated protocol to minimize the risk of unblinding and rigorous angina and medications assessment through 5 years of follow-up. Demonstrating long-term angina reduction would certainly mark one point in favor of BRSs. However, harder clinical benefits need to be noted after bioresorption to justify the current enthusiasm toward this technology.[19]

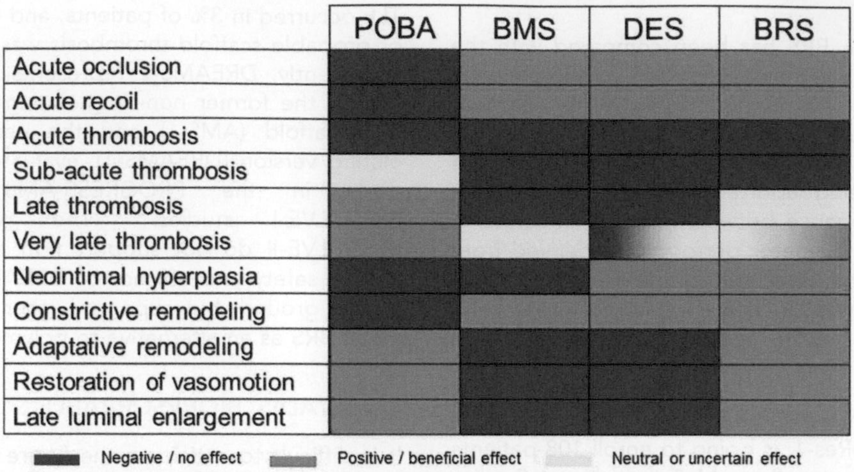

	POBA	BMS	DES	BRS
Acute occlusion				
Acute recoil				
Acute thrombosis				
Sub-acute thrombosis				
Late thrombosis				
Very late thrombosis				
Neointimal hyperplasia				
Constrictive remodeling				
Adaptative remodeling				
Restoration of vasomotion				
Late luminal enlargement				

▬▬ Negative / no effect   ▬▬ Positive / beneficial effect   ▬▬ Neutral or uncertain effect

Fig. 1. Putative comparison of plain old balloon angioplasty (POBA), bare-metal stents (BMS), drug-eluting stents (DES), and bioresorbable scaffolds (BRS) based on noncomparative data.

Although the future of BRSs is uncertain, the present is not clearer. Patients with BRSs currently represent only a minority of patients undergoing PCI in high-traffic catheterization laboratories in Europe.[2] PCI with BRSs can be more demanding than with DESs if the lesion complexity increases, and may require more resources to obtain a perfect result (ie, time, balloons for predilation, intravascular imaging).[2] Overall, BRSs are less forgiving technologies than DESs, and the importance of a flawless technique cannot be overlooked with these devices, particularly because thrombotic events have so far mostly reported in the periprocedural period, implying a role for suboptimal procedures.[20] One might ask, "Who is thrombogenic, the scaffold or the doctor?"[21] The answer stays in the middle.

Doctors should realize that implanting current-generation BRSs implies a commitment toward a potential long-term benefit. If ongoing studies show this to be true, then patients certainly deserve the additional care and skill that are required to implant BRSs. If this is not the case, then the entire matter needs reassessment. However, BRSs serve as an example of how history repeats itself. First-generation DESs were also not exempt from technical shortcomings and safety issues. The advent of second-generation DESs is a good example of how industry efforts can be impactful in ameliorating clinical outcomes. In this scenario, several companies are currently trying to enter the BRS market: the many differentiating characteristics of their investigational devices (including time of resorption, radial strength, and strut thickness) make this endeavor of notable interest.

There is no doubt that such competition will exert positive effects on the quality, safety, and efficacy of BRS technologies in general.

SUMMARY

BRSs have been enthusiastically heralded as the fourth revolution in interventional cardiology, after the advent of plain old balloon angioplasty, bare-metal stents, and DESs. Current evidence with the Absorb device supports noninferiority to second-generation DESs in selected and relatively simple lesions. However, meta-analyses have recently raised concerns about a higher rate of device thrombosis compared with second-generation DESs. Ongoing studies will clarify if this limitation is offset by long-term benefits of BRSs. In parallel, industry efforts are devoted to make these devices more user-friendly and safer in the early term.

REFERENCES

1. Byrne RA, Serruys PW, Baumbach A, et al. Report of a European Society of Cardiology-European Association of Percutaneous Cardiovascular Interventions task force on the evaluation of coronary stents in Europe: executive summary. Eur Heart J 2015;36(38):2608–20.

2. Tamburino C, Latib A, van Geuns RJ, et al. Contemporary practice and technical aspects in coronary intervention with bioresorbable scaffolds: a European perspective. EuroIntervention 2015; 11(1):45–52.

3. Iqbal J, Onuma Y, Ormiston J, et al. Bioresorbable scaffolds: rationale, current status, challenges, and future. Eur Heart J 2014;35(12):765–76.

4. Puricel S, Arroyo D, Corpataux N, et al. Comparison of everolimus- and biolimus-eluting coronary stents with everolimus-eluting bioresorbable vascular scaffolds. J Am Coll Cardiol 2015;65(8):791–801.

5. Diletti R, Serruys PW, Farooq V, et al. ABSORB II randomized controlled trial: a clinical evaluation to compare the safety, efficacy, and performance of the Absorb everolimus-eluting bioresorbable vascular scaffold system against the XIENCE everolimus-eluting coronary stent system in the treatment of subjects with ischemic heart disease caused by de novo native coronary artery lesions: rationale and study design. Am Heart J 2012;164(5):654–63.

6. Serruys PW, Chevalier B, Dudek D, et al. A bioresorbable everolimus-eluting scaffold versus a metallic everolimus-eluting stent for ischaemic heart disease caused by de-novo native coronary artery lesions (ABSORB II): an interim 1-year analysis of clinical and procedural secondary outcomes from a randomised controlled trial. Lancet 2015;385(9962):43–54.

7. Sabate M, Windecker S, Iniguez A, et al. Everolimus-eluting bioresorbable stent vs. durable polymer everolimus-eluting metallic stent in patients with ST-segment elevation myocardial infarction: results of the randomized ABSORB ST-segment elevation myocardial infarction-TROFI II trial. Eur Heart J 2015;37(3):229–40.

8. Kimura T, Kozuma K, Tanabe K, et al. A randomized trial evaluating everolimus-eluting Absorb bioresorbable scaffolds vs. everolimus-eluting metallic stents in patients with coronary artery disease: ABSORB Japan. Eur Heart J 2015;36(47):3332–42.

9. Gao R, Yang Y, Han Y, et al. Bioresorbable vascular scaffolds versus metallic stents in patients with coronary artery disease: ABSORB China trial. J Am Coll Cardiol 2015;66(21):2298–309.

10. Ellis SG, Kereiakes DJ, Metzger DC, et al. Everolimus-eluting bioresorbable scaffolds for coronary artery disease. N Engl J Med 2015;373(20):1905–15.

11. Cassese S, Byrne RA, Ndrepepa G, et al. Everolimus-eluting bioresorbable vascular scaffolds versus everolimus-eluting metallic stents: a meta-analysis of randomised controlled trials. Lancet 2016;387(10018):537–44.

12. Capodanno D, Gori T, Nef H, et al. Percutaneous coronary intervention with everolimus-eluting bioresorbable vascular scaffolds in routine clinical practice: early and midterm outcomes from the European multicentre GHOST-EU registry. EuroIntervention 2015;10(10):1144–53.

13. Lipinski MJ, Escarcega RO, Baker NC, et al. Scaffold thrombosis after percutaneous coronary intervention with ABSORB bioresorbable vascular scaffold: a systematic review and meta-analysis. JACC Cardiovasc Interv 2016;9(1):12–24.

14. Verheye S, Ormiston JA, Stewart J, et al. A next-generation bioresorbable coronary scaffold system: from bench to first clinical evaluation: 6- and 12-month clinical and multimodality imaging results. JACC Cardiovasc Interv 2014;7(1):89–99.

15. Haude M, Ince H, Abizaid A, et al. Safety and performance of the second-generation drug-eluting absorbable metal scaffold in patients with de-novo coronary artery lesions (BIOSOLVE-II): 6 month results of a prospective, multicentre, non-randomised, first-in-man trial. Lancet 2016;387(10013):31–9.

16. Erbel R, Di Mario C, Bartunek J, et al. Temporary scaffolding of coronary arteries with bioabsorbable magnesium stents: a prospective, non-randomised multicentre trial. Lancet 2007;369(9576):1869–75.

17. Waksman R, Erbel R, Di Mario C, et al. Early- and long-term intravascular ultrasound and angiographic findings after bioabsorbable magnesium stent implantation in human coronary arteries. JACC Cardiovasc Interv 2009;2(4):312–20.

18. Haude M, Erbel R, Erne P, et al. Safety and performance of the drug-eluting absorbable metal scaffold (DREAMS) in patients with de-novo coronary lesions: 12 month results of the prospective, multicentre, first-in-man BIOSOLVE-I trial. Lancet 2013;381(9869):836–44.

19. Byrne RA. Bioresorbable vascular scaffolds: will promise become reality? N Engl J Med 2015;373(20):1969–71.

20. Capodanno D, Joner M, Zimarino M. What about the risk of thrombosis with bioresorbable scaffolds? EuroIntervention 2015;11(Suppl V):V181–4.

21. Colombo A, Ruparelia N. Who is thrombogenic: the scaffold or the doctor? back to the future! JACC Cardiovasc Interv 2016;9(1):25–7.

Design and Comparison of Large Vessel Stents

Balloon Expandable and Self-Expanding Peripheral Arterial Stents

Sandeep M. Patel, MD[a,b], Jun Li, MD[a,b], Sahil A. Parikh, MD[a,b,*]

KEYWORDS

- Endovascular stenting • Stent design • Balloon expandable stent • Self-expanding stent

---

KEY POINTS

- Vascular injury with balloon angioplasty and endovascular stent implantation induces neointimal hyperplasia and results in clinical restenosis.
- Endovascular stent design and engineering impact clinical performance and influences the vascular response to injury.
- Restenosis remains a vexing problem in endovascular intervention requiring adaptation of principles of stent design from balloon expandable to self expanding stents due to the need for peripheral stents to have greater elasticity.
- Optimization of stent design has led to novel approaches to modulating the vascular response to injury and improving the hemodynamic and rheological impact of stenting with clinical improvements in stent performance.
- Continued evolution of stent design and engineering will hopefully yield improved clinical outcomes in more demanding peripheral vascular applications.

BACKGROUND

The origin of the word "stent" hails from Charles Thomas Stent, a London dentist who created Stent's compound to fill the empty space inside the root of a tooth.[1] The word was subsequently adapted into the surgical and urologic world to describe a substance that holds a graft in place or, in reference to intraluminal use, to maintain patency.[1]

Although the concept of arterial stenting was first described by Drs Charles Dotter and Melvin Judkins in 1964, it was not until 1983 that the word "stent" was used in the literature to describe the use of an endoluminal coil stent.[1,2] Thereafter, Dr Julio Palmaz developed the balloon-expandable (BX) Palmaz stent in 1985, and Drs Ulrich Sigwart and Jacques Puel developed the self-expanding (SX) Wallstent in 1987. Since then, stents have been widely adopted for revascularization of a wide variety of vascular beds.

Due to its widespread use in critical vascular territories, the mechanical and biologic performance of a stent is crucial. Some important parameters of stent performance include deliverability, ease of deployment, and long-term patency. In all forms of endovascular stenting, angioplasty occurs concomitantly with stent implantation and produces vessel injury by way of plaque disruption, endothelial denudation, disruption of the intima media, and thrombus formation. This injury activates the stereotypical cascade of the vascular response to injury ultimately resulting in subsequent neointimal proliferation and adverse remodeling. Stents were

---

[a] Department of Medicine, Case Western Reserve University School of Medicine, Cleveland, OH 44106, USA;
[b] Division of Cardiovascular Medicine, Harrington Heart and Vascular Institute, University Hospitals Case Medical Center, 11100 Euclid Avenue, Cleveland, OH 44106, USA
* Corresponding author.
E-mail address: Sahil.Parikh@UHhospitals.org

Intervent Cardiol Clin 5 (2016) 365–380
http://dx.doi.org/10.1016/j.iccl.2016.03.005
2211-7458/16/$ – see front matter © 2016 Elsevier Inc. All rights reserved.

introduced as a way to prevent abrupt vessel closure and to reduce late lumen loss as discussed elsewhere in this issue (See Elmore JB, Mehanna E, Parikh SA, et al: Restenosis of the Coronary Arteries: Past, Present, Future Directions). However, stent implantation results in not only an immediate but also a chronic vascular injury, resulting in vigorous and prolonged neointimal proliferation.[3] Long-term patency rates are driven by several factors, including procedural components, such as acute tissue injury and stent expansion, and pharmacologic determinants, such as stent-bound antiproliferative drugs and systemic antiplatelet inhibition. However, underpinning all of these aspects is the fundamental design of the bare metal scaffold itself.

Endovascular stenting has evolved over the last 50 years since its inception into the framework of management of vascular atherosclerotic disease. Stent design has evolved as lesion complexity has increased. Nevertheless, certain first principles regarding stent design have been recapitulated time and again with every new iteration of endovascular stents. This article reviews the principles of endovascular stent design (Fig. 1),[4] and compares and contrasts key aspects of BX and SX stents.

STENT DESIGN: PHYSICAL PROPERTIES

At the crux of stent design is the balance of clinical characteristics and performance. As one attribute improves, it is typically at the expense of another attribute. First, a clear understanding of four basic physical properties is important to conceptualize the engineering of stents: (1) yield stress, (2) tensile strength, (3) Young's modulus of elasticity, and (4) strain. The static properties of stent material include yield stress and tensile strength, whereas the dynamic properties include Young's modulus and strain.[5] Since the ratio of force to unit area defines stress, thus yield stress refers to the ability of a metal to undergo a specific stress until it deforms irreversibly (plastic deformation). At the other extreme is tensile strength, which is the highest level of stress a material can withstand before it fails or fractures. Strain is the amount of deformation a material can undergo for a unit of given stress. If stress and strain are plotted, the slope of the line is referred to Young's modulus of elasticity (Fig. 2). The stiffer the material, the larger the modulus because there is less deformation per unit of stress. A complex interplay between the stent composition including metal and polymeric components and these physical properties allows for optimization of stent deliverability, performance, and lifespan (Table 1).

STENT DESIGN: THREE-DIMENSIONAL PROPERTIES

The three-dimensional (3D) construction of an endoluminal stent results in three additional design parameters that can be modified to alter stent performance: (1) radial resistive force, (2) chronic outward force (COF), and (3) hoop

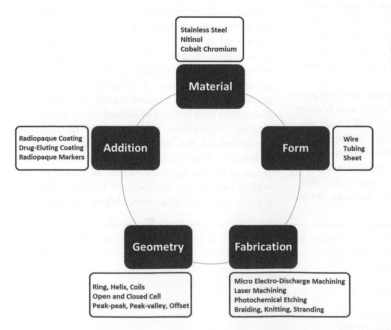

Fig. 1. The five pillars of stent engineering. (*Adapted from* Sangiorgi G, Melzi G, Agostoni P, et al. Engineering aspects of stents design and their translation into clinical practice. Ann Ist Super Sanita 2007;43:90.)

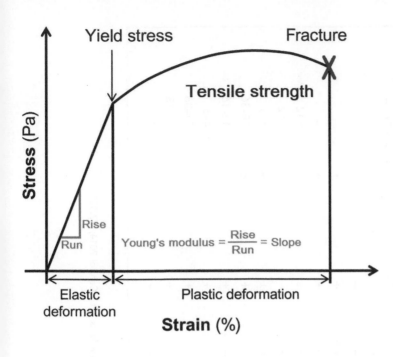

Fig. 2. Stress/strain relationship. A graphic representation of the stress and strain relationship. Note that all metallic stents are bound by Young's modulus of elasticity until they reach the Yield Stress point that results in permanent stent deformity. Further stress and strain upon the stent after reaching the Yield Stress point results in reaching Tensile or Ultimate Strength and is the representation of the maximum level of stress that the stent can be subjected to prior to fracture. (*Adapted from* Tambaca J, Canic S, Kosor M, et al. Mechanical behavior of fully expanded commercially available endovascular coronary stents. Tex Heart Inst J 2011;38:491–501)

strength.[5] Radial resistive force and COF are specific to SX stents, whereas hoop strength applies to BX stents (Fig. 3).

Hoop strength, the 3D counterpart of yield stress, is the amount of compressive force needed to collapse a BX stent. The interplay of hoop strength and Young's modulus is important in producing an easy to expand, structurally sound stent after deployment. Balloon expansion results in dilation of a crimped stent, creating plastic deformation of the stent in a predictable fashion. The greater the modulus, the more pressure is necessary to expand the stent. Conversely, the greater the modulus, the more resistance there is to any external recoil produced by the vessel itself, maintaining the ability of the stent to scaffold a vessel.

For SX stents, superelasticity and "shape-memory" are required to help facilitate expansion and prevent collapse. Superelasticity and "shape-memory" allow for a metal to undergo a greater degree of elastic deformation before reaching the yield point of irreversible deformation, thus these alloys frequently demonstrate a very low Young's modulus and a very high yield stress. Nitinol, an alloy of nickel and titanium, is predominantly used for SX stents because its physical properties can be manipulated based on the environmental temperature, known as martensitic transformation (Fig. 4).[5] The term radial resistive force is used to describe the amount of resistance the stent can impart against an external compressive force that is trying to collapse the stent. In the case of SX

stents, this varies based on the amount of oversizing that is done and the vessel recoil that occurs after expansion.[5] COF is the force exerted by the SX stent on the vessel wall as it expands to its nominal size, which helps afford stability against the vessel lumen and prevents downstream migration generated by bloodstream shear stress (Fig. 5).[5] This property, unique to SX stents, may produce damaging effects over time because it causes persistent unopposed vessel expansion and sustained deep vessel injury.

STENT DESIGN: HEMODYNAMICS AND FLOW MODIFICATION

The mere presence of an endovascular stent illicits a multitude of biological responses that induce inflammation, thrombosis, neo-intimal proliferation, and re-endothelialization. The summation of these events alters the flow and hemodynamics of the normal vessel.[6]

Normal arterial flow is governed by two fundamental laws: conservation of mass and conservation of momentum (Navier-Stokes equations).[6] As arterial blood flows through a vessel a physical interaction between blood and endothelial cells occurs. Due to circulatory flow pressure upon the vessel wall, wall shear stress is generated, which represents the product of blood viscosity and wall shear rate (the spatial gradient between the blood velocity and the wall).[7] It is the presence of low wall shear stress that dictates regions that are most

Table 1
Various metallic alloys and bioabsorbable polymers and their physical properties

Material	Density (g/cm³)	Elastic Young's Modulus (Gpa)	Tensile Strength (Mpa)	Elongation at Break (%)	Corrosion Resistance	Visibility	Biocompatibility	Low Recoil	Biodegradability (mo)
316L SS	8	193	670	48	+	+	+	+	–
L-605 (CoCr)	9.1	243	>1000	>50	+	+	+	+	–
MP-35N (CoCr)	8.43	233	930	45–60	+	+	+	+	–
PtCr	9.9	203	834	45	+	++	+	+	–
Nitinol	6.45	40	800–1200	12–25	+	+	+	+	–
Pure iron	7.8	150	210	40	–	+	±	+	>12
Fe-35MN	7.6	235	530	32	–	+	–	n/a	>12
WE43 (Mg)	1.83	40–130	280	6.8	–	+	±	+	1–3
PLLA	1.2–1.4	2.7–4.0	40–65	2–6[a]	n/a	–	+	±	18–36
PDLA	1.8	1.0–3.5	40–55	2–6[a]	n/a	–	+	±	12–16
PGA	1.5	6.0–7.0	90–110	1–2[a]	n/a	–	+	±	4–6
PCL	1.1	0.2–0.4	25–35	>300[a]	n/a	–	+	±	24–36
PLGA (85 L/15G)	1.3	2.0–4.0	40–70	2–6[a]	n/a	–	+	±	12–18
PDLGA (50 DL/ 50G)	1.2–1.3	2.0–4.0	40–50	1–4[a]	n/a	–	+	±	1–2

Abbreviations: n/a, not applicable.
[a] Indicative value for raw material.
Data from Foin N, Lee RD, Torii R, et al. Impact of stent strut design in metallic stents and biodegradable scaffolds. Int J Cardiol 2014;177:805.

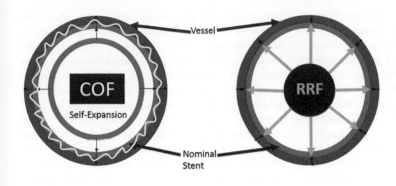

Fig. 3. Properties of self-expanding stents. Chronic outward force (COF) represents the force that a nominally expanded stent applies to the vessel wall as a manifestation of continued expansion (represented by the *yellow line*). Radial resistive force (RRF) represents the force that can be applied to the stent by the vessel itself, and is the manifestation of the stent's ability to resist compression.

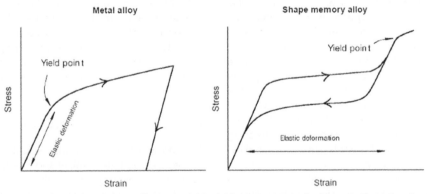

Fig. 4. Stress/strain relationships of metallic versus nitinol (shape memory alloy) stents. Note that in nitinol stents, the relationship plateaus because of the elasticity of nitinol as compared to metal. (*From* Whittaker DR, Fillinger MF. The engineering of endovascular stent technology: a review. Vasc Endovascular Surg 2006;40:91; with permission.)

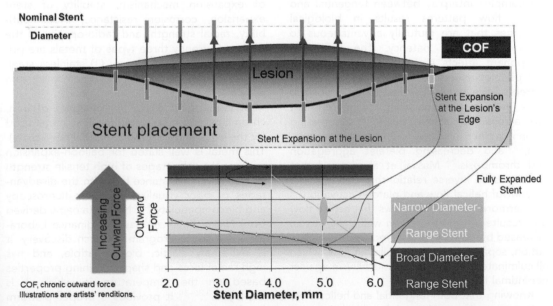

Fig. 5. Graphic representation of COF after stent deployment as a function of stent diameter range. Note that COF is present in all self-expanding stents but the narrower the diameter range the steeper the COF curve.

vulnerable to atherosclerosis.[7–9] In fact, based on the most current theory of hemodynamics and atherosclerosis, the lower the wall stress, the lower the uniform alignment of endothelial cells with the direction of blood flow resulting in atherosclerosis-prone regions.[10] In addition to regions of low wall stress, regions of disturbed flow cause zones of flow re-circulation, flow separation, non-uniform stress, and stagnation that all contribute to endothelial cell down-regulation of anti-thrombotic mechanisms,[11,12] while simultaneously causing the expression of pro-coagulant molecules, which in turn result in platelet adhesion and thrombosis.[13–15]

Understanding the complex interplay of flow modification, wall shear stress, and endothelial cell function is key to grasping the fundamental basis for the effects of stent implantation and their long-term effects and outcomes on local hemodynamics. One further key is to recognize the contribution of the heart in generating secondary flow patterns, thus complicating the tangential, straight-line, parabolic flow that would be present in an ex vivo model of peripheral arterial flow. The torsional and twisting forces that occur with systole and diastole allow for a more effective contraction and emptying of blood into the aorta.[16–18] This spiral contraction results in a clockwise systolic rotation and a counterclockwise diastolic rotation in the abdominal aorta beyond the renal arteries.[19] This helical flow has been shown to be present in iliac and femoral arteries via Doppler ultrasonography and phase contrast MRI.[20–22] In fact, the complex interplay between tangential and helical flow patterns results in biological outcomes that are mutually advantageous to maintaining vessel patency. The tangential component affects endothelial cell alignment and platelet adhesion,[19] while the helical flow patterns have been observed to be a positive force in terms of enhancing oxygen/nutrient flux across the arterial wall,[23,24] suppressing luminal surface oxidized-lipoprotein concentration,[25] and decreasing platelet aggregation and thrombosis.[26] Massai et al. showed that there was an inverse relationship between the amount of helical flow and platelet activation.[14] Furthermore, Caro et al. shows that helical flow also resulted in more uniform wall shear stress, increased blood flow mixing, reduced flow stagnation, separation, and instability in flow, which all culminated in a protective mechanism against neointimal hyperplasia.[27]

Knowing that both tangential and helical flow patterns are present in peripheral arteries, one can begin to understand the complexities that occur with the disruption of these in vivo flow patterns after stent implantation. In addition to stent contact with endothelium that results in local injury patterns as dictated by cell design and strut characteristics as delineated below, local and downstream hemodynamics are altered by each individual strut in the form of proximal and distal recirculation zones.[28] The disruption of spiral and tangential flow resulting in flow stagnation results in a reduction of wall shear stress with the associated cascade as discussed above.[12,29] Further, stents are typically "sized" to the vessel wall, where there is the inherent possibility of over- or under-sizing.[30] Over-sizing results in a reduction in blood flow velocity and decreases wall shear stress within the stent and produces "step-up" regions at the ends of the stent that cause flow re-circulation. Under-sizing may leave a gap between the stent and the arterial wall that increase flow resistance and increases wall shear stress.[12,30]

STENT DESIGN: ALLOYS AND CORROSION

The materials used for endovascular stents must possess several mechanical and chemical characteristics to ensure proper delivery, deployment, and biocompatibility. The metals used in the production of stents have been evolving as the science of metallurgy advances. Chemically, endovascular stents should exhibit minimal corrosion. In the case of metallic stents, the choice of metal affects the deliverability, type of expansion mechanism, stability of stent expansion, corrosion resistance, biocompatibility, radial strength, and radio-opacity of the device. Currently three types of metals are primarily used in stent design: (1) stainless steel, (2) nitinol, and (3) cobalt or platinum chromium alloy (see Table 1).[31]

Stainless steel 316L, an amalgam of iron, chromium, and nickel, was the first metal used for the initial endovascular stent (Palmaz-Schatz). This metal is well suited for balloon-expansion and has the advantages of high tensile strength and corrosion resistance but with the disadvantages of poor visualization under fluoroscopy and biocompatibility.[3,32] Nitinol (a name derived from Nickel Titanium Naval Ordinance Laboratory) is a space program research discovery. It is extremely elastic, biocompatible, and has high radial force and shape-retaining properties based on the temperature in which it is deployed.[3,32–34] It provides a proper platform for SX stents. Cobalt and platinum chromium stents tend to be thinner but retains adequate radial strength and radio-opacity because of higher tensile strength (see **Table 1**).[34,35]

Corrosion occurs as a function of the amount of chloride content in the surface layer of the stent.[5] The reaction between the environment and the stent metal is mitigated by the presence of a surface oxide layer that protects the underlying structure from further corrosive degradation.[5] Depending on the alloy used, the surface oxide protective layer varies and so does its breakdown potential. In metallurgy, the resting potential of a certain alloy must be lower than the breakdown potential as supported by the thin surface oxide protection layer. For instance, stainless steel (type 304) has no difference in either potential making, it very susceptible to corrosion and breakdown, whereas titanium has almost a nine-fold difference in resting and breakdown potentials resulting in high resistance to breakdown.[5] However, nitinol does not have a great deal of corrosion resistance, because the formation of a superficial oxidized layer alters the release of nickel into the surrounding tissue. This can provoke local inflammation and induce expression of cellular adhesion molecules linked with tissue proliferation, clinical restenosis, and reduced long-term stent patency.[5] Thus corrosion, choice of metal used, and the formation of a protective surface oxide layer may also impact the biologic response to endovascular stent placement.

STENT DESIGN: ASSOCIATED MATERIALS

The use of additional synthetic and natural graft material attached to the outer aspect of stents as seen in stent grafts or covered stents results has also been attempted to improve stent performance. However, this covering can induce its own inflammatory reaction. Abluminal neointimal growth is advantageous to prevent stent migration, but if neointimal proliferation encroaches on the vascular lumen, thrombosis and clinical restenosis can occur. Experimentally, studies have shown that after 6 weeks of polyester-covered and uncovered-nitinol stents in canine aortas, the patency and flow hemodynamics were no different between the two types of stents, but an increase in neointimal hyperplasia was seen in the covered grafts. Similar events were noted in other stent-grafts when compared to uncovered stents.[36,37] A detailed review of large vessel stent grafts is provided elsewhere in this issue (See Powell A, Kashyap VS: Design and Clinical Considerations for Endovascular Stent Grafts).

STENT DESIGN: COATINGS

Chemical stent coatings have been used to help enhance biocompatibility and improve the interaction between the stent, cells, and molecules present in the stent environment.[34] An extensive review on the impact of surface modification on stent biocompatibility is reviewed elsewhere in this issue. (See Kolandaivelu K, Rikhtegar F: The Systems Biocompatibility of Coronary Stenting).

STENT DESIGN: RADIO-OPACITY

With existing technology, the successful deployment of a stent is based in part on the ability of the operator to visualize the stent using fluoroscopic guidance. The radio-opacity of the metal varies with type of alloy used. Stainless steel is more radiopaque than nitinol, but both are difficult to image fluoroscopically. To improve visibility, highly radiopaque markers made from gold, platinum, or tantalum can be added to the ends of the stent via sleeves around the struts, rivets integrated in a strut, or welded-on tabs. Electroplating with gold is being used to enhance visibility; however, it may produce issues on other imaging modalities, such as computed tomography or MRI, which results in flare or scatter artifacts at the sites of metallic stent struts affecting the imaging characteristics of the other aspects of the image. In a more contemporary view, the use of MRI protocols for stent positioning and deployment may be a future prospect for percutaneous therapies and thus a nickel-titanium compound may be more suitable for such endeavors because it produces fewer artifacts.

STENT DESIGN: FABRICATION

BX and SX stents are typically made from wires, tubes, or sheet metal. The method of fabrication is typically based on the material used for production. Wires can be molded into a helical shape or take the form of multiple, independent rings that are bound or welded together. Tubular and sheet designs are etched by way of laser, chemically, or electrically. These designs use links to connect adjoining rings. Laser cutting is used to produce a majority of vascular stents and are most effective at producing intricate patterns to optimize flexibility, deliverability, and crimping. However, in laser etching, a heat-affected zone is produced that needs to be removed to improve the performance of the stent. To prevent this issue, novel methods of cutting and etching have been developed, including water-jet cutting and photochemical etching.

STENT DESIGN: GEOMETRY

The importance of stent geometry cannot be underestimated. Stent geometry dictates many of the delivery properties of the stent delivery system; however, more importantly it contributes to the acute and chronic performance of the stent.[38,39] Importantly, geometry has been shown to impact overall vessel healing and endothelial function post stent deployment, thus underpinning the critical importance of stent engineering.[40] Most stent designs in the initial days of development were slotted-tubes (Palmaz-Schatz) or coil-based (Gianturco-Roubin Flex) platforms. Five main stent geometries are typically used in present day manufacturing (Fig. 6).

Individual Rings

These are Z-shaped rings that are single elements not used for vascular application. These rings are sutured to graft material for support of the endoprosthesis.

Sequential Rings

Comprised of both struts (expandable Z-shaped elements, also known as crests) and nodes (connecting elements or connectors), the sequential ring design is the basis for most vascular stents. The intricacies of the sequential ring design are exemplified by the representative illustration in Fig. 6. The base composition consists of multiple series of struts or rings that are attached by connectors. The rings can either be in-phase (peak-peak), out-of-phase (peak-valley), or offset peak-to-peak depending on placement of the connectors. Because of the variety of possible connections between struts and nodes, resultant cells are produced that dictate stent performance. Regular connections imply a node at every inflection point, while periodic connection alternate between nodes and free struts. The number of connectors determines the balance between flexibility and scaffolding. The quantity and configuration of connectors between adjacent rings distinguish so-called "open" and "closed" cell stents. If all adjacent rings are connected together, this typically constitutes a "closed" cell design, whereas if some or all of the adjacent rings are not connected, that represents an "open" cell design. The primary advantage of a closed-cell design is to allow for more uniform scaffolding of the stented segment regardless of the degree of bending, but it may reduce overall stent flexibility. In contrast, an open-cell design allows fewer internal inflection points and connections to bridging elements, thus allowing for less vessel scaffolding but often greater flexibility.

The orientation of struts (ie, peak-peak, peak-valley, or offset peak-to-peak) determines several important characteristics. The peak-valley conformation yields the smallest degree of stent shortening when it is expanded beyond its nominal diameter. The peak-peak conformation offers excellent durability and scaffolding but at a cost of decreased flexibility and deliverability. The addition of various flexible bridging connectors (U-, V-, S-, and N-shaped) allows adjacent rings to accommodate to the vessel architecture while maintaining structural integrity (Fig. 7).

The number of crests and bar arm length help dictate the maximum expansion range, a trait

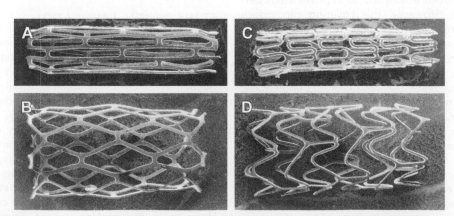

Fig. 6. Scanning electron photomicrographs of stents of different configurations. Slotted tube stent before (A) and after (B) expansion; corrugated ring stent before (C) and after (D) expansion (original magnification ×100). (From Rogers C, Edelman ER. Endovascular stent design dictates experimental restenosis and thrombosis. Circulation 1995;91(12):2995–3001; with permission.)

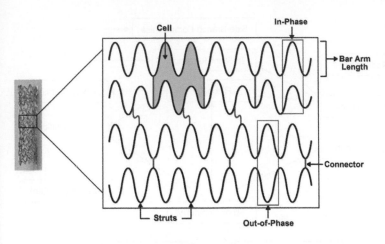

Fig. 7. Stent nomenclature. Struts and connectors form the backbone of a stent. Struts can be in-phase (peak-peak) or out-of-phase (peak-valley) as illustrated, or may be offset peak-to-peak. These components play a vital role in the overall performance of a stent.

that determines how much a stent can be over-expanded before losing its structural integrity and scaffolding becomes compromised. This loss of physical integrity is sometimes referred to as "ringing out" of a stent. A larger expansion range is achieved by either increasing the number of struts or extending the bar arm length.

Woven

Typically used for SX stents, this type of design uses braided strands of wire. These stents produce excellent coverage, but may shorten during expansion. Radial strength of this stent depends on axial fixation of the proximal and distal ends of the stent, but tends to be very high.[5]

Helical

This design of stent is based on a helical spiral that has minimal or no internal connections that allows for the highest degree of flexibility and lowest level of longitudinal support. Limitations are related to elongation and compression during deployment, which results in irregular cell size.[5]

Coil

Coil stents, similar to that used by Dotter in 1983, are extremely flexible but impractical because of the lack of radial and axial strength, coupled with low acute gain and high late loss and rate of restenosis.[34,41] Because of the coil configuration, a low-expansion ratio results in high-profile devices making them difficult to deliver. These have limited applications in present day endovascular procedures.

STENT DESIGN: STRUT THICKNESS

A variety of stent strut thicknesses have been studied. Ultimately, the fundamental width of

the struts have differing effects. Thinner struts may incorporate more deeply into the arterial wall and cause less angulation and stretching of the arterial wall.[41] Although thicker struts result in greater radio-opacity and radial force for improved arterial support, the larger struts result in abnormal apposition, greater arterial injury, and neointimal proliferation. Previous studies have demonstrated an absolute increase in restenosis in thick-strut stents.[42] Extrapolating from coronary arterial disease trials, the ISAR-STEREO series demonstrated that strut thickness greater than or equal to 140 μm was associated with 10% absolute increase in the angiographic restenosis rate ($P = .003$) and a follow-up series demonstrated that this result was independent of stent geometry.[43,44]

STENT DESIGN: NUMBER OF STRUTS

The number of stent struts supporting the vessel affects the cross-sectional polygonal configuration of the stent. It has been previously reported that having more than 12 struts around the 360° arc of a vascular lumen results in less vascular injury and mural thrombus formation than in a design with fewer struts in which there is more angulation and deeper arterial injury. However, a study demonstrating 1:1 sizing of the stent to the artery regardless of the number struts results in less neointimal hyperplasia than with vascular overstretch.[38]

STENT DESIGN: FLEXIBILITY, TRACKING, AND CONFORMABILITY

Stent flexibility, tracking, and conformability are determined based on the stent alloy, geometry, and strut design. These are secondary characteristics that are the result of the interplay of the basic stent design elements (**Fig. 8**). Flexibility

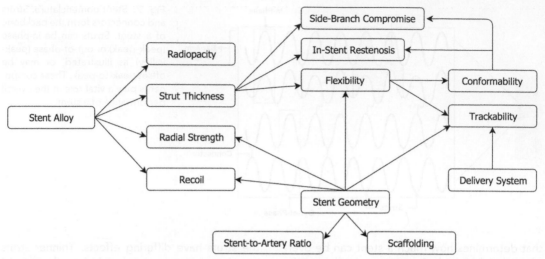

Fig. 8. The interplay of stent characteristics. (*From* Price MJ, Mosley WJI. Fundamentals of drug-eluting stent design. In: Price MJ, editor. Coronary stenting: A companion to Topol's textbook of interventional cardiology. Philadelphia: Elsevier Saunders; 2014:238; with permission.)

refers to the force required to bend the stent to a specific radius and in turn affects the tracking, which describes the ease at which a stent can be advanced to the target lesion. Tracking is quantified by the amount of work required to pass a stent through tortuosity. Finally, conformability describes the characteristic of a stent to adapt to the natural curvature of the vessel without resulting in kinking of the vessel.[45] Although secondary characteristics, these are pivotal stent design considerations that are at the forefront of stent implantation and delivery.

STENT DESIGN: RADIAL AND LONGITUDINAL STRENGTH

The construct of a stent is subjected to radial and longitudinal forces that may result in suboptimal acute results or late lumen loss over time. Radial strength as mentioned above is the compressive resistance force of a stent to maintain its diameter and the vessel lumen after implantation. The radial strength is imperative to the treatment of ostial lesions and highly calcific lesions where diameter maintenance over time is critical.[45] Longitudinal strength is the compressive resistance against shortening or elongation when exposed to pushing or pulling. Ormiston et al. have demonstrated that fewer connectors between stent segments results in lower longitudinal strength and more susceptibility to longitudinal compression,[46] which occurs particularity during in vivo situation such as post-dilation, distal stenting, or the use of imaging catheters.

STENT DESIGN: DRUGS AND DELIVERY

Drug delivery is a large component of the management of peripheral arterial disease. For more details on stent-based drug delivery (See Tzafriri AR, Edelman ER: Endovascular Drug Delivery and Drug Elution Systems: First principles; and Habib A, Finn AV: Anti-Proliferative Drugs for Restenosis Prevention, in this issue). Three platforms for stent drug delivery are used in the modern era: (1) metallic stents with drug bound to the surface of the stent, (2) metallic stents with an outer-layer of polymer that is drug-loaded, and (3) a bioabsorbable polymeric stent that is loaded with a slowly eluting drug. Metallic stents with polymeric coating loaded with drug make up the bulk of the current generation of stents. Homogeneous drug delivery requires uniform stent expansion and strut spacing. Thus, stent designs are pivotal for predictable drug delivery and to avoid either subtherapeutic or toxic levels of drug in the vascular wall.

Local drug delivery requires three essential components: (1) consistent delivery of the agent at therapeutic doses, (2) maintenance of intramural drug concentrations long enough to affect pathophysiologic processes, and (3) little or no drug toxicity. With the delivery of the drug, the retention of intramural drug is a function of specific binding of drug to the components of the vascular wall. A more detailed consideration of stent-based drug delivery is discussed elsewhere in this issue. However, because there is no other consideration of peripheral arterial drug-eluting stents (DES), we briefly review the clinical results of DES used in the peripheral vasculature.

Bare Metal Versus Drug-eluting Peripheral Stents

Durability of stenting has been the limitation of bare metal stents (BMS) in peripheral arterial disease. To advance the field, the pattern of stenting in coronary artery disease has been followed by advancing from bare metal to drug-eluting platforms.

The SIROCCO trial was the first randomized, controlled trial to evaluate the use of sirolimus-eluting stent compared with BMS (SMART Stent, Cordis, Johnson & Johnson, Miami Lakes, FL) in approximately 93 patients (50% in each cohort) that demonstrated that the 2-year in-stent restenosis and target lesion revascularization rates were not significantly different between the two cohorts.[47] Dake and colleagues followed approximately 7 years later with the Zilver PTX trial comparing polymer free paclitaxel-eluting stents (n = 236) with angioplasty with provisional BMS (n = 238).[48] Interestingly, the trial established that the 2-year event-free survival, primary patency, and overall clinical benefit were higher with paclitaxel-eluting stents compared with angioplasty ± BMS.[49]

Although these trials were designed for femoropopliteal disease, there continues to be a patency benefit with endovascular stent-based drug delivery in the infrapopliteal vessels. A 2013 meta-analysis of four randomized controlled trials and two observational studies concluded that 1-year outcomes, which included primary patency, freedom from target lesion revascularization, and clinical improvement, were superior for DES compared with BMS (DES, n = 287; BMS, n = 257).[50] Specifically,

sirolimus has been studied in two randomized controlled trials in 2012. Bosiers and colleagues[51] demonstrated that angiographic restenosis and vessel patency were significantly improved with DES (n = 99) compared with angioplasty alone (n = 101), whereas no statistically significant difference was noted in clinically driven target vessel revascularization or index-limb amputation. The findings were recapitulated in the ACHILLES trial with the use of a Cypher Select stent (Cordis, Johnson & Johnson, Bridgewater, NJ).[52] In contrast, Rastan and colleagues[53] found that event-free survival and target vessel revascularization were improved in the setting of sirolimus-eluting stents (n = 82) compared with BMS (n = 79).

STENT DEPLOYMENT

Stents are manufactured with all of the previously mentioned properties in mind, but classification can be simplified into two major subtypes: SX and BX (Table 2).

Balloon-Expandable

BX stents are crimped over a balloon and expanded via balloon inflation. BX stents are resistive of expansion but are inelastic, which is in contrast to SX stents and thus compress if enough external pressure is applied. As such, BX stents are typically used in vessels with little extrinsic compression, such as visceral, iliac, and proximal infrapopliteal vessels. Because of the issue of radial stiffness, a BX stent is approximately three times stiffer than a similar SX stent, and thus reduces overall vessel compliance compared with an SX stent. BX engineering has attempted to use thin, flexible struts and nodes, which allow for longitudinal flexibility and conformability to

---

Table 2
Properties of balloon-expandable and self-expanding stents

	Balloon-Expandable Stent	**Self-Expanding Stent**
Production	Made in the crimped state Delivery balloon loaded inside stent	In the nominal diameter Crimped into a smaller diameter and housed within a delivery sheath
Lesion preparation	Direct stenting is common Predilation not necessary	Predilation is mandatory
Delivery	Resists balloon expansion Recoils after balloon deflation	Assist vessel expansion No recoil after balloon deflation
Longevity	Will become smaller in diameter over time	Proper oversizing leads to chronic outward force to expand vessel
Response to external force	After critical external pressure is exceeded, collapse/buckling Irreversible without subsequent repeat dilation	Elastically recoil after flattening No strength limitations

the vessel; however, BX stents are still inferior in this respect compared with SX stents. BX stents seems to recoil after balloon deflation because of the external forces applied by the vessel. A major disadvantage of BX stents is that the diameter of the stent seems to decrease over time, but because of engineering advances newer generation BX stents can overcome this recoil. Neointimal hyperplasia may result and BX stents continue to remain near the intima, thus any hyperplasia indicates a constriction of the lumen and stent.[42] Deliverability of a BX stent is determined by the integration of the stent and balloon profile, which taken together are called the stent delivery system. Because balloon inflation results in stent deployment, accuracy of placement is high. Given that BX stents are deployed with balloons and at higher pressure, the deployment itself results in vessel expansion.

Efficacy of BX stenting compared with angioplasty for peripheral arterial disease has been evaluated in multiple clinical trials. A 2008 meta-analysis assessing a pooled primary patency rate at 1 year in a total of seven randomized trials (N = 452 patients) demonstrated that angioplasty was not significantly different than BX stenting (angioplasty, 45%–84%; BX, 63%–90%; $P = .962$).[54] A second meta-analysis done by a different group (N = 614 limbs in 519 patients) in which angioplasty and BX stenting was performed in 291 limbs found that primary patency at 6 months did favor BX stenting over angioplasty alone ($P<.05$), but found no difference at 12 months.[55]

Self-Expanding

The Wallstent (Boston Scientific, Marlborough, MA) represents a prototypical SX stent that is not made of nitinol. In any case, the SX stents have relatively no strength limitation and elastically recover even after complete flattening or crushing. This makes SX stents very suitable for superficial locations in the carotids, superficial femoral, and proximal popliteal arteries. Secondarily, SX stents are not susceptible to lack of radial strength and thus stent design is focused on optimizing other design elements. SX stents are radially compliant and remain more conformable to the vessel shape to avoid high contact forces at the ends of the stent. The recoil of an SX stent is quite significant compared with BX stents and thus is not preferred in coronary and renal architecture. However, a properly sized SX stent applies continued COF to expand the vessel after deployment and after about 1 month, BMS SX stents have been incorporated into the vascular

wall of the vessel and hyperplasia is the norm. The SX stent supports the vessel from the outer portion of the vessel lining and continues to expand to support the vessel wall rather than allowing another surface to be in contact with the blood. The overall delivery profile is based on the strut dimensions (width) and deliverability is similar to BX stents (although traditionally inferior). However, a major difference is that SX stents are completely housed in delivery catheters that need to be "unsheathed" to place and deliver the SX stent. SX stents do not have enough stiffness and outward force to dilate a calcific lesion and thus predilation or postdilation is necessary.

Clinical outcomes of contemporary SX stents have been evaluated. In the DURABILITY I study, the Protégé EverFlex (ev3 Inc, Plymouth, MN), a SX nitinol stent, was studied in 151 patients with femoropopliteal arterial disease and demonstrated that the primary patency rate at 1 year was 72% with a stent fracture rate of less than 10%.[56] The RESILIENT trial randomized 206 patients with femoropopliteal disease to the LifeStent (Bard Peripheral Vascular Inc, Tempe, AZ) versus angioplasty with provisional stenting. At 1 year, patency was 81% compared with 37% in the angioplasty cohort.[57] Similar findings were seen in the SUMMIT registry (EPIC stent, Boston Scientific, Marlborough, MA) and the COMPLETE SE study (Medtronic Vascular, Santa Rosa, CA) both of which demonstrated 1-year primary patency rates between 73% and 85%.[58,59] Armstrong and colleagues[60] demonstrated in 254 patients that nitinol SX stents compared with balloon angioplasty has similar performance in terms of 1-year primary patency if femoropopliteal lesions were less than or equal to 150 mm, whereas those with greater than or equal to 150-mm lesions, 1-year patency outcomes were 34% (stenting) versus 49% (angioplasty) ($P = .006$), even when multiple stents are used.

The Zilver PTX (Cook Medical, Bloomington, IN) is a paclitaxel-coated nitinol SX DES that was compared against provisional stenting with the drug-coated or BMS stent.[48] A total of 236 patients had implantation of the Zilver PTX, whereas 238 patients underwent percutaneous transluminal angioplasty. One hundered-twenty patients had angioplasty failure and were randomized 1:1 BMS to DES. The primary patency rate was 83% in the Zilver PTX cohort compared with 33% in the angioplasty group. Furthermore, in the provisional cohort, DES was also superior to BMS (90% to 73% primary patency).[48] Geraghty and colleagues[61] randomized patients with femoropopliteal disease and claudication in the VIBRANT study to either BMS SX stents or a Viabahn stent, a PTFE material reinforced with nitinol scaffolding (WL Gore and Associates, Newark, DE) that demonstrated no significant difference in primary patency at 3 years between the two cohorts; however, the rate of stent fracture was extremely low (2.6%) in the Viabahn cohort as compared with the traditional nitinol BMS SX stent (50%).

Vascular Mimetic

While BX and SX stents have transformed the management of peripheral arterial disease, the need for stent platforms that withstand extension/contraction, torsional, compression, flexion stressors while maintaining patency and reducing the risk of stent fractures has been a gap that has not been filled. However, the recently FDA approved Supera peripheral stent system (Abbott Vascular, Santa Clara, CA) provides a new development in SX technology (Fig. 9). As a woven SX stent that uses six pairs of nitinol wires arranged in a helical pattern, the Supera system has a proprietary deployment system that allows stent stacking in certain lesion locations to provide increased degree of support where necessary. Retrospective registry data confirms that among femoro-popliteal lesions the one and 2-year primary patency rates were 83–85% and 62–76%, respectively, depending on length of lesion.[62] Furthermore, three independent retrospective studies found no stent fractures in approximately 200 patients.

In addition to Supera, other biomimetic devices are currently under investigation. For instance, it has been well established that neo-intimal hyperplasia results in regions of low shear stress. Flow mechanics in peripheral arteries typically demonstrate a helical pattern that allows for elevated wall shear and reduction of atherosclerosis and intimal hyperplasia.[7,8,63,64] A recently developed helical stent known as Bio-Mimics 3D (Veryan Medical Ltd., Horsham, UK) was studied in the MIMICS trial. The stent design is cut from a nitinol tube and has a 3D helical geometry that is laser cut and self-expanding (Fig. 10). Novel to the design, the stent allows for the gradual reduction of radial force to

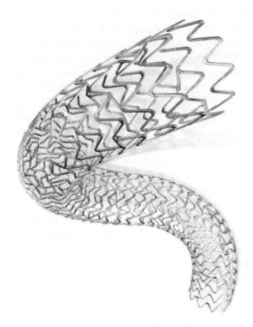

Fig. 10. Helical stent 3D modeling of the BioMimics 3D helical stent design that allows for increased levels of shear stress preventing neo-intimal hyperplasia.

improve the transition from stent to artery on either side of the stent which reduces "step-up" phenomenon and decreases stent fracture at sites of increased shortening due to bending. The overall purpose of the stent was to allow for continued elevation of wall shear while providing a smooth, non-disruptive transition between artery and stent that distributes compressive strain forces across the entire length of the stent preventing kinking, fracture, recirculation, stagnation, while promoting high wall shear stress, that results in improved long-term patency Fifty helical stents and 26 non-helical, standard stents were studied in a 2:1 randomized fashion and the trial demonstrated that primary patency was improved with the helical design (72% vs 55%), in addition to being superior with regards to freedom from clinically driven re-intervention.[65] This trial was preliminary in terms of safety and patency assessment, however, does generate significant evidence that mimetic devices attempting to model arterial hemodynamics may provide superior results with further development.

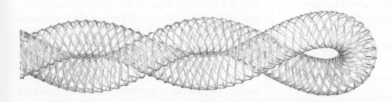

Fig. 9. Supera stent illustration of the interwoven nitinol wires that allow for flexibility and long-term patency of the Supera stent.

The Perfect Stent

The concept of the design of a "perfect" stent continues to evolve. Based on the above design characteristics, the ideal stent must be able to achieve short and long-term success. In the metallic stent, regardless of either SX or BX, first principles of stent design need to be abided by. The stent should be deliverable, fluoroscopically visible, conform to the vessel architecture, induce minimal vascular trauma, maintain scaffold integrity and minimize restenosis, prevent plaque prolapse, have a low incidence of fracture, have a low corrosion capacity, and uniformly deliver drug (should it be a DES) to reduce neointimal hyperplasia, while avoiding local drug toxicity.[45,66] To date, no single stent has been able to achieve all of the above characteristics simultaneously, however, with the advent of vascular mimetics, we are one step closer to modeling vascular anatomy and hemodynamics. Engineering trade-offs in design continue to limit the ability of the "perfect" stent due to conflicts between hemodynamic laboratory testing and in vitro performance. In any case, the future appears bright with respect to better designs, improved performance, and excellent short and long-term outcomes.

SUMMARY

Since the introduction of balloon angioplasty, interventionalists have struggled with target lesion restenosis. Tremendous advances in stent engineering and understanding of the biology underlying restenosis have led to significant improvements in vessel patency rates. Nonetheless, restenosis still remains challenging, particularly in the lower extremities where endovascular stents are subject to a unique array of forces and stressors not present in other vascular beds. Optimization of stent performance is to achieve the ideal balance between successful delivery/deployment and long-term patency. Stent design remains a pivotal and evolving science, whereby ongoing advancements will continue to pave the way for improvement in clinical outcomes.

REFERENCES

1. Roguin A. Stent: the man and word behind the coronary metal prosthesis. Circ Cardiovasc Interv 2011; 4:206–9.
2. Dotter CT, Buschmann RW, McKinney MK, et al. Transluminal expandable nitinol coil stent grafting: Preliminary report. Radiology 1983;147: 259–60.
3. Lau KW, Mak KH, Hung JS, et al. Clinical impact of stent construction and design in percutaneous coronary intervention. Am Heart J 2004; 147:764–73.
4. Sangiorgi G, Melzi G, Agostoni P, et al. Engineering aspects of stents design and their translation into clinical practice. Ann Ist Super Sanita 2007; 43:89–100.
5. Whittaker DR, Fillinger MF. The engineering of endovascular stent technology: a review. Vasc Endovascular Surg 2006;40:85–94.
6. Kokkalis E, Aristokleous N, Houston JG. Haemodynamics and flow modification stents for peripheral arterial disease: a review. Ann Biomed Eng 2016; 44:466–76.
7. Caro CG. Discovery of the role of wall shear in atherosclerosis. Arterioscler Thromb Vasc Biol 2009;29:158–61.
8. Caro CG, Fitz-Gerald JM, Schroter RC. Arterial wall shear and distribution of early atheroma in man. Nature 1969;223:1159–60.
9. Caro CG, Fitz-Gerald JM, Schroter RC. Atheroma and arterial wall shear. Observation, correlation and proposal of a shear dependent mass transfer mechanism for atherogenesis. Proc R Soc Lond B Biol Sci 1971;177:109–59.
10. Malek AM, Alper SL, Izumo S. Hemodynamic shear stress and its role in atherosclerosis. JAMA 1999; 282:2035–42.
11. Chien S. Effects of disturbed flow on endothelial cells. Ann Biomed Eng 2008;36:554–62.
12. Murphy EA, Boyle FJ. Reducing in-stent restenosis through novel stent flow field augmentation. Cardiovasc Eng Technol 2012;3:353–73.
13. Bassiouny HS, Song RH, Kocharyan H, et al. Low flow enhances platelet activation after acute experimental arterial injury. J Vasc Surg 1998;27: 910–8.
14. Massai D, Soloperto D, Gallo D, et al. Shear-induced platelet activation and its relationship with blood flow topology in a numerical model of stenosed carotid bifurcation. Eur J Mech B/Fluids 2012;35:92–101.
15. Varga-Szabo D, Pleines I, Nieswandt B. Cell adhesion mechanisms in platelets. Arterioscler Thromb Vasc Biol 2008;28:403–12.
16. Buckberg GD. Basic science review: the helix and the heart. J Thorac Cardiovasc Surg 2002;124: 863–83.
17. Kocica MJ, Corno AF, Carreras-Costa F, et al. The helical ventricular myocardial band: global, three-dimensional, functional architecture of the ventricular myocardium. Eur J Cardiothorac Surg 2006; 29(Suppl 1):S21–40.
18. Torrent-Guasp F, Ballster M, Buckberg GD, et al. Spatial orientation of the ventricular muscle band: physiologic contribution and surgical

implications. J Thorac Cardiovasc Surg 2001;122: 389–92.

19. Frazin LJ, Vonesh MJ, Chandran KB, et al. Confirmation and initial documentation of thoracic and abdominal aortic helical flow. An ultrasound study. ASAIO J 1996;42:951–6.

20. Harloff A, Albrecht F, Spreer J, et al. 3d blood flow characteristics in the carotid artery bifurcation assessed by flow-sensitive 4d mri at 3t. Magn Reson Med 2009;61:65–74.

21. Stonebridge PA, Brophy CM. Spiral laminar flow in arteries? Lancet 1991;338:1360–1.

22. Caro CG, Doorly DJ, Tarnawski M, et al. Non-planar curvature and branching of arteries and n on-planar-type flow. Proc R Soc 1996;452:185–97.

23. Liu X, Fan Y, Deng X. Effect of spiral flow on the transport of oxygen in the aorta: a numerical study. Ann Biomed Eng 2010;38:917–26.

24. Morbiducci U, Ponzini R, Rizzo G, et al. Mechanistic insight into the physiological relevance of helical blood flow in the human aorta: an in vivo study. Biomech Model Mechanobiol 2011;10: 339–55.

25. Ding Z, Fan Y, Deng X, et al. Effect of swirling flow on the uptakes of native and oxidized ldls in a straight segment of the rabbit thoracic aorta. Exp Biol Med (Maywood) 2010;235:506–13.

26. Zhan F, Fan Y, Deng X. Swirling flow created in a glass tube suppressed platelet adhesion to the surface of the tube: its implication in the design of small-caliber arterial grafts. Thromb Res 2010;125: 413–8.

27. Caro CG, Cheshire NJ, Watkins N. Preliminary comparative study of small amplitude helical and conventional eptfe arteriovenous shunts in pigs. J R Soc Interface 2005;2:261–6.

28. Jimenez JM, Davies PF. Hemodynamically driven stent strut design. Ann Biomed Eng 2009;37: 1483–94.

29. Wentzel JJ, Gijsen FJ, Schuurbiers JC, et al. The influence of shear stress on in-stent restenosis and thrombosis. EuroIntervention 2008;4(Suppl C): C27–32.

30. Chen HY, Hermiller J, Sinha AK, et al. Effects of stent sizing on endothelial and vessel wall stress: potential mechanisms for in-stent restenosis. J Appl Physiol (1985) 2009;106:1686–91.

31. Foin N, Lee RD, Torii R, et al. Impact of stent strut design in metallic stents and biodegradable scaffolds. Int J Cardiol 2014;177:800–8.

32. Bertrand OF, Sipehia R, Mongrain R, et al. Biocompatibility aspects of new stent technology. J Am Coll Cardiol 1998;32:562–71.

33. Lau KW, Johan A, Sigwart U, et al. A stent is not just a stent: stent construction and design do matter in its clinical performance. Singapore Med J 2004;45: 305–11 [quiz: 312].

34. Hara H, Nakamura M, Palmaz JC, et al. Role of stent design and coatings on restenosis and thrombosis. Adv Drug Deliv Rev 2006;58:377–86.

35. Alicea LA, Aviles JI, López IA, et al. Mechanics biomaterials: stents. Course Materials in the Department of General Engineering, University of Puerto Rico, Mayaguez. 2004.

36. Avino A, Johnson B, Bandyk D, et al. Does prosthetic covering of nitinol stents alter healing characteristics or hemodynamics? J Endovasc Ther 2000;7:469–78.

37. Cejna M, Virmani R, Jones R, et al. Biocompatibility and performance of the wallstent and the wallgraft, jostent, and hemobahn stent-grafts in a sheep model. J Vasc Interv Radiol 2002;13:823–30.

38. Garasic JM, Edelman ER, Squire JC, et al. Stent and artery geometry determine intimal thickening independent of arterial injury. Circulation 2000; 101:812–8.

39. Sullivan TM, Ainsworth SD, Langan EM, et al. Effect of endovascular stent strut geometry on vascular injury, myointimal hyperplasia, and restenosis. J Vasc Surg 2002;36:143–9.

40. Rogers C, Parikh S, Seifert P, et al. Endogenous cell seeding. Remnant endothelium after stenting enhances vascular repair. Circulation 1996;94: 2909–14.

41. Moscucci M. Grossman & baim's cardiac catheterization, angiography, and intervention. Philadelphia (PA): Lippincott Williams & Wilkins; 2013.

42. Rogers C, Tseng DY, Squire JC, et al. Balloon-artery interactions during stent placement: a finite element analysis approach to pressure, compliance, and stent design as contributors to vascular injury. Circ Res 1999;84:378–83.

43. Kastrati A, Mehilli J, Dirschinger J, et al. Intracoronary stenting and angiographic results: strut thickness effect on restenosis outcome (isar-stereo) trial. Circulation 2001;103:2816–21.

44. Pache J, Kastrati A, Mehilli J, et al. Intracoronary stenting and angiographic results: strut thickness effect on restenosis outcome (isar-stereo-2) trial. J Am Coll Cardiol 2003;41:1283–8.

45. Price MJ, Mosley WJI. Fundamentals of drug-eluting stent design. In: Price MJ, editor. Coronary stenting: a companion to topol's textbook of interventional cardiology. Philadelphia (PA): Elsevier Saunders; 2014. p. 238.

46. Ormiston JA, Webber B, Webster MW. Stent longitudinal integrity bench insights into a clinical problem. JACC Cardiovasc Interv 2011;4: 1310–7.

47. Duda SH, Bosiers M, Lammer J, et al. Drug-eluting and bare nitinol stents for the treatment of atherosclerotic lesions in the superficial femoral artery: long-term results from the sirocco trial. J Endovasc Ther 2006;13:701–10.

48. Dake MD, Ansel GM, Jaff MR, et al. Paclitaxel-eluting stents show superiority to balloon angioplasty and bare metal stents in femoropopliteal disease: twelve-month zilver ptx randomized study results. Circ Cardiovasc Interv 2011;4:495–504.

49. Dake MD, Ansel GM, Jaff MR, et al. Sustained safety and effectiveness of paclitaxel-eluting stents for femoropopliteal lesions: 2-year follow-up from the zilver ptx randomized and single-arm clinical studies. J Am Coll Cardiol 2013;61:2417–27.

50. Antoniou GA, Chalmers N, Kanesalingham K, et al. Meta-analysis of outcomes of endovascular treatment of infrapopliteal occlusive disease with drug-eluting stents. J Endovasc Ther 2013;20: 131–44.

51. Bosiers M, Scheinert D, Peeters P, et al. Randomized comparison of everolimus-eluting versus bare-metal stents in patients with critical limb ischemia and infrapopliteal arterial occlusive disease. J Vasc Surg 2012;55:390–8.

52. Scheinert D, Katsanos K, Zeller T, et al. A prospective randomized multicenter comparison of balloon angioplasty and infrapopliteal stenting with the sirolimus-eluting stent in patients with ischemic peripheral arterial disease: 1-year results from the achilles trial. J Am Coll Cardiol 2012;60:2290–5.

53. Rastan A, Brechtel K, Krankenberg H, et al. Sirolimus-eluting stents for treatment of infrapopliteal arteries reduce clinical event rate compared to bare-metal stents: long-term results from a randomized trial. J Am Coll Cardiol 2012;60:587–91.

54. Mwipatayi BP, Hockings A, Hofmann M, et al. Balloon angioplasty compared with stenting for treatment of femoropopliteal occlusive disease: a meta-analysis. J Vasc Surg 2008;47:461–9.

55. E Y, He N, Wang Y, et al. Percutaneous transluminal angioplasty (PTA) alone versus pta with balloon-expandable stent placement for short-segment femoropopliteal artery disease: a metaanalysis of randomized trials. J Vasc Interv Radiol 2008;19: 499–503.

56. Bosiers M, Torsello G, Gissler HM, et al. Nitinol stent implantation in long superficial femoral artery lesions: 12-month results of the durability i study. J Endovasc Ther 2009;16:261–9.

57. Laird JR, Katzen BT, Scheinert D, et al. Nitinol stent implantation versus balloon angioplasty for lesions in the superficial femoral artery and proximal popliteal artery: twelve-month results from the resilient randomized trial. Circ Cardiovasc Interv 2010;3: 267–76.

58. Werner M, Piorkowski M, Thieme M, et al. Summit registry: one-year outcomes after implantation of the epic self-expanding nitinol stent in the femoropopliteal segment. J Endovasc Ther 2013;20:759–66.

59. Laird JR, Jain A, Zeller T, et al. Nitinol stent implantation in the superficial femoral artery and proximal popliteal artery: twelve-month results from the complete se multicenter trial. J Endovasc Ther 2014;21:202–12.

60. Armstrong EJ, Saeed H, Alvandi B, et al. Nitinol self-expanding stents vs. Balloon angioplasty for very long femoropopliteal lesions. J Endovasc Ther 2014;21:34–43.

61. Geraghty PJ, Mewissen MW, Jaff MR, et al. Three-year results of the vibrant trial of viabahn endoprosthesis versus bare nitinol stent implantation for complex superficial femoral artery occlusive disease. J Vasc Surg 2013;58:386–95.e4.

62. Garcia L, Jaff MR, Metzger C, et al. Wire-interwoven nitinol stent outcome in the superficial femoral and proximal popliteal arteries: twelve-month results of the superb trial. Circ Cardiovasc Interventions 2015;8.

63. Coppola G, Caro C. Arterial geometry, flow pattern, wall shear and mass transport: potential physiological significance. J R Soc Interf 2009;6: 519–28.

64. Carlier SG, van Damme LC, Blommerde CP, et al. Augmentation of wall shear stress inhibits neointimal hyperplasia after stent implantation: Inhibition through reduction of inflammation? Circulation 2003;107:2741–6.

65. Zeller T. Mimics. VIVA Physicians Symp. 2014.

66. Wholey MH, Finol EA. Designing the ideal stent. Endovascular Today 2007;25–34.

Design and Clinical Considerations for Endovascular Stent Grafts

Alexis Powell, MD, Vikram S. Kashyap, MD*

KEYWORDS

- Abdominal aortic aneurysm (AAA) • EVAR • Endograft • Aortic neck • Active fixation
- Radial force

KEY POINTS

- Endovascular treatment for aortic abnormality is an excellent alternative option for patients who are not good candidates for conventional open surgery.
- The evolution of the stent-graft design has been an exercise in expanding indications for use, safety, and miniaturization.
- The most important limitations to overcome are achieving high-quality aortic neck "healthy" landing zone, smaller diameter delivery systems, and endografts that allow for more angled aortic necks.
- New endovascular techniques were developed to accommodate endovascular repair of abdominal aortic aneurysms falling outside the above criteria in patients deemed poor open candidates.

INTRODUCTION

Aortic aneurysms are localized dilatations of the arterial wall and most commonly affect the infrarenal abdominal aorta. Abdominal aortic aneurysm (AAA) has a multifactorial pathology, with both environmental and genetic risk factors. Occlusive atherosclerotic disease, smoking, male gender, and hypertension are known risk factors for aneurysmal degeneration. Genetic predisposition gives a relative risk of 1.9 in people with a family history.[1]

AAAs develop typically without symptoms and are commonly found incidentally on imaging for unrelated symptoms. The natural history of aneurysms is to gradually expand silently over time, and unfortunately, can commonly rupture without warning or symptoms; this often results in hemodynamic compromise and death. Aortic aneurysm rupture carries a mortality of greater than 80%, with a traditional 50% in hospital

mortality after open repair.[2] Current recommendations advocate intervention for AAAs greater than 5.5 cm in diameter, symptomatic aneurysms, or ruptured.

Traditional open surgical repair uses a large intra-abdominal or retroperitoneal incision, followed by replacement of diseased aorta with prosthetic graft. The operation requires general anesthesia and is commonly associated with significant morbidity and mortality.

Endovascular treatment of aortic abnormality is an excellent alternative option for patients who are not good candidates for conventional open surgery. Multiple studies have demonstrated endovascular aortic aneurysm repair (EVAR) as an alternative to open surgery with lower perioperative morbidity and mortality, and overall long-term outcomes that rival the traditional repair. In recent years, the design of these stent grafts has evolved to adapt to

---

Department of Vascular Surgery and Endovascular Therapy, University Hospitals Case Medical Center, 11100 Euclid Avenue, Cleveland, OH 44106, USA
* Corresponding author.
E-mail address: Vikram.Kashyap@uhhospitals.org

Intervent Cardiol Clin 5 (2016) 381–389
http://dx.doi.org/10.1016/j.iccl.2016.03.003
2211-7458/16/$ – see front matter © 2016 Elsevier Inc. All rights reserved.

more and more challenging aortic abnormality and anatomic constraints.

Historically, the endovascular stent graft is associated primarily for treatment of AAAs, although they are being used more and more to treat many other different types of aortic abnormality—including dissection, atherosclerotic disease, pseudoaneurysm, and aortic trauma/transection. In addition, the grafts are now used for aneurysms of other arteries, including the thoracic aorta and iliac arteries.

THE FIRST ENDOVASCULAR AORTIC ANEURYSM REPAIRS

Dr Nicholas Volodos and Dr Juan Carlos Parodi are credited for developing the first aortic endografts. Dr Volodos did so in the 1970s to 1980s era and developed a fabric-covered Z-stent, tested in animal models. First implantation in a human aorta was on March 24, 1987 for treatment of a traumatic thoracic aortic aneurysm. Also in 1987, Volodos and colleagues[3] performed the first EVAR in a human.

Endovascular repair of AAAs in the Western hemisphere was simultaneously underway and was initially described by Parodi and colleagues,[4] who performed their first successful EVAR in 1990. Their idea for a device initially came from coronary stenting and utilization of similar stents on a larger-size scale for the aorta.

Finally, Dr Timothy Chuter designed, made, and used the first modern-day bifurcated stent graft for AAA, the first modular system for endovascular repair of an aortic arch aneurysm, and the first modular system for bilateral iliac aneurysms.[5]

OVERVIEW OF ENDOVASCULAR AORTIC ANEURYSM REPAIR TECHNIQUE

Although the technique of placing endovascular stent grafts has evolved since the first grafts, the basic principles remain the same. Access to the aorta is typically achieved via common femoral artery access in the groin, and fluoroscopic imaging is used to identify the anatomy of the abdominal aorta. The Seldinger technique is used to introduce catheters, sheaths, and delivery system of the stent graft into place into the aorta over a guidewire, and the endograft is deployed into position. Following complete delivery of the endograft components, a seal is achieved using balloon angioplasty at both the proximal and the distal landing zones of "healthy" aorta, excluding the aneurysm sac from circulation.

DESIGN PRINCIPLES OF ENDOVASCULAR STENT GRAFTS

The evolution of the stent-graft design has been an exercise in expanding indications for use, safety, and miniaturization.

Original designs for endovascular aortic aneurysm exclusion devices are somewhat similar to those of today. In fact, most follow many of the same design principles—metal skeleton with graft fabric material. The early stent-graft devices were modified balloon-mounted stents sutured to a Dacron tube graft. These devices were delivered through a sheath, and the balloon-mounted stent was deployed in the neck of the aneurysm.[4] Early stent-graft designs were limited in scope of treatment, with a unibody design, and would require additional cross-femoral bypass if the aneurysm involved the aortic bifurcation or the iliac arteries.

Soon after their publication in the early 1990s, there were many modifications to the original design, including the introduction of the bifurcated stent graft designed by Dr Chuter and colleagues,[6] introduction of aortic fixation via metallic barbs and the use of self-expanding Nitinol stents for proximal fixation. Early designs and devices were based on physician modification of readily available components to create an endograft. Soon after the introduction and initial reports of success, the design of the devices was taken over by industry and underwent rapid evolution and multiple alterations.

One of the 2 first commercially available stent grafts relied on passive fixation to keep the stent graft in place as well as seal the aneurysm. Passive fixation required radial force from the stent structure pressing outward on the wall of the infrarenal aorta. In order to accomplish this, stent grafts require oversizing beyond the aortic neck diameter. This technique has been questioned in the past[7] and more recently with the introduction of gel polymer proximal seal stent grafts.[8,9] It has been hypothesized that oversizing grafts creates increased outward forces that, over time, may induce further conformational degenerative changes in the aortic wall. Isolated passive fixation devices have now largely been phased out of current use.

Although the other of the first 2 US Food and Drug Administration (FDA) -approved, commercially available grafts did use active hooks for fixation, it was fraught with problems that ultimately led to its discontinuation. Most currently available grafts use active fixation techniques in their stent grafts via metal barbs that are designed to penetrate the aortic wall and hold the stent graft in place. This fixation system increases the disconnection or "pull-out" force required and thus decreases the risk of migration. Current stent-graft manufacturers are quick to note the distinction between fixation and seal. Seal still requires oversizing and the radial forces inherent to each graft to ensure restriction of flow around the graft at the neck of the aneurysm.

As time progressed, product delivery systems have also been seen to shrink significantly in diameter. This shrinkage can be largely attributed to the evolution of components used in the systems—metal alloy skeleton and graft material. Obviously, the purpose of this is to allow for use in a larger spectrum of patients with smaller anatomy that previously was thought impossible for endovascular stenting. For example, the first-generation EVAR devices typically were 22- to 24 French in profile, even up to a 27-French outer-diameter profile. Up until 2010, most EVAR devices were still greater than 20 French in profile. Currently, most manufacturers offer devices in the 18-, 16-, and even 14-French profile. Cook Zenith low-profile AAA devices use 16- or 17-French profile, whereas Cook Zenith uses 18- to 22-French sheaths. Gore Excluder main device uses an 18- or 20-French sheath. Medtronic Endurant can be delivered "bareback", and the delivery system measures 18 or 20 French, depending on diameter of the graft. The Cook Zenith fenestrated device is deployed through a 20- to 22-French delivery sheath.

Over time, various metal alloys have supplanted the use of stainless steel as the skeleton of endografts. Although some manufacturers continue to use stainless steel partially in design, most have moved toward nickel titanium alloy (Nitinol) or cobalt chromium alloy as the scaffold for the stent grafts. As compared with stainless steel and cobalt chromium, nitinol has several advantages in its biomechanical design. Nitinol exhibits significantly more elasticity than the previously mentioned materials.[10,11] Specifically, stainless steel and cobalt chromium exhibit low elastic deformation as compared with nitinol (nitinol more closely follows the deformation characteristics of the various tissues of the living body). Whichever stent skeleton is used, it must be a balance of strength, light weight, and compressibility to maximize graft durability, while allowing for minimal delivery system diameter.

Graft material has also contributed to the decrease in delivery size. Similar to open aneurysm repair technology, endograft material options primarily are polytetrafluoroethylene (PTFE, or Teflon) or polyethylene terephthalate (PET, synthetic polyester Dacron). PTFE is an inert material that biochemically consists of a carbon-fluorine polymer chain, discovered in 1938 by Roy Plunkett and patented 3 years later. The fluorine creates a shield around the carbon backbone, making it impermeable to blood.[12] It also has thermal stability and chemical resistance.

PET (Dacron polyester) also is considered to have both good biocompatibility and chemical resistance. It is a rigid plastic material that is woven or knitted. It is a very porous material that originally required "preclotting" intraoperatively to contain blood. Now, modern PET grafts are impregnated with one of a few biomaterials to make them less porous—including gelatin, collagen, or albumin. Multiple studies have demonstrated that PET grafts induce a greater inflammatory response than PTFE grafts.[13,14] Almost all current aortic endografts are PTFE or woven polyester.

CLINICAL AND ANATOMIC CONSIDERATIONS/LIMITATIONS

Early EVAR devices were generally limited to straightforward proximal neck anatomy. The indications for use for most early devices were limited to the following guidelines regarding proximal neck anatomy[15]:

1. Neck length of 15 mm
2. Neck diameter between 17 and 25 mm
3. Aortic neck angulation of less than 45°or less
4. 10% to 20% oversizing

CURRENT ENDOVASCULAR STENT GRAFTS COMMERCIALLY AVAILABLE (IN THE UNITED STATES)

Table 1 lists all currently available, FDA-approved endovascular grafts.

MODERN ADVANCES: PARALLEL STENTS, FENESTRATED ENDOVASCULAR ANEURYSM REPAIR, AND OTHER NEW DEVICES

New endovascular techniques were developed to accommodate endovascular repair of AAAs falling outside the above criteria in patients deemed poor open candidates. Thanks to the initial work of Greenberg and colleagues,[16] the most limiting factor of "neck length" below the renal arteries has become an almost obsolete requirement through the use of parallel

Table 1
Currently available, US Food and Drug Administration–approved endovascular grafts

Endograft	Materials Graft/Support	Suprarenal Fixation	Active Proximal Barbs	Native Aortic Neck Diameter (mm)	Native Iliac Diameter (mm)	Main Device Delivery Sheath Diameter (French)	Potential Advantages
AneuRx (Medtronic)	Polyester/nitinol	No	No	20–26	8–22	21	Hydrophilic delivery system
Endurant (Medtronic)	Polyester/electropolished nitinol	Yes	Yes	19–32	8–25	20	Indications include short (10 mm) aortic neck, angulated neck
Powerlink (Endologix)	PTFE/cobalt chromium alloy	Yes	No	18–32	10–23	17	Anatomic fixation at iliac bifurcation, low profile
Excluder (Gore)	PTFE/nitinol	No	Yes	19–29	10–18.5	20	C3 delivery system, ability to recapture and reposition body
Talent (Medtronic)	Polyester/nitinol	Yes	No	18–32	8–22	24	Indication for short (10 mm) aortic neck, angulated necks
Zenith (Cook Medical)	Polyester/stainless steel	Yes	Yes	18–32	8–20	26	Spiral Z flexible limbs
Zenith fenestrated (Cook Medical)	Polyester/stainless steel	Yes	Yes	19–31	9–21	20	Juxtarenal aneurysm
Ovation (Trivascular)	PTFE/nitinol	Yes	Yes	16–30	8–20	15	Low-profile, proximal sealing ring
Aorfix (Lombard)	PTFE/nitinol	No	Yes	19–29	8–19	22	Flexibility, angulated neck

stent grafts. The next most challenging criterion to overcome was a high degree of angulation. Thanks to the work by the Lombard Company, new grafts have reached the market that have extended the degree of neck angulation to 90° or less.

Parallel stent grafting has allowed vascular surgeons to march proximally on the abdominal aorta, even into the thoracic aorta, to repair various abnormalities involving branch vessels. These adjunct stents are placed between the aortic wall and endograft, effectively increasing the neck length by raising the ostium of the renal artery.[17] Since its initial implementation, many have expanded on and further defined the snorkel-and-chimney technique.

Fenestrated endovascular grafts are similar in construction to their nonfenestrated counterpart as far as construction, that is, PTFE fabric, nitinol stents, suprarenal barbs, although they include fenestrations or scallops in the fabric through which renovisceral vessels will be perfused (Fig. 1). Center-line imaging is used to "straighten out" the aorta and aneurysm to mimic in vivo stiff wires; precise measurements of the native aorta diameter and locations of the visceral vessels are marked (Fig. 2). In addition, "clock positions" are used to measure angulation of visceral vessels for fenestration and scallop placement on the graft (Fig. 3). Once the grafts are created to the specific requirements of each individual patient, the grafts are deployed at the appropriate cranial-caudal level oriented such that the fenestrations align with the assigned visceral vessel. The visceral vessels are cannulated from within the lumen of the main-body stent graft, and stents are

placed through the main body into the branch vessel to preserve flow.

Unlike parallel stent grafts, these visceral stents are in series with the main body, obtaining blood flow from the lumen of the stent graft, not the proximal or distal native aorta. These grafts are special ordered and constructed tailored to patient-specific anatomy. Anatomic limitations of these grafts are determined after careful review by biomechanical engineers, because there are certain distances required between each fenestration, scallop, and the proximal and distal edges of the graft in order to maintain outward radial force required for graft stability.

Fenestrated cases show a preference for less angulated renal vessels with shorter renal artery cannulation times, fluoroscopy times, and overall procedural duration. In contrast, snorkel EVAR cases showed more favorable findings when there was greater downward angulation to the renal vessels.[18] Fenestrated cases involve cannulation of visceral vessels from within the lumen of the main-body stent graft after deployment of enough graft material to free a visceral ostium from the stent graft. Cannulation of the visceral vessels in these cases occurs from a more caudal arterial bed; therefore, less downward angulation theoretically makes it easier for the surgeon to cannulate the visceral ostium. On the other hand, snorkel cases have visceral cannulation occur from a more proximal arterial bed with cannulation occurring in a cranial to caudal direction. In this situation, downward angulation theoretically aids in visceral cannulation.[19]

Antegrade deployment of parallel stent grafts for preservation of aortic side-branches when treating aneurysmal disease has shown excellent patency. In the largest reported series of snorkel repairs with a mean follow-up of 17 months, primary patency was 94%, with secondary patency of 95.3%. Type Ia endoleak was present in 5.7% with secondary intervention rates of 37.9%. Overall survival of patients in this high-risk cohort for open repair at latest follow-up was 79%.[20] This 2015 registry data show improved outcomes as compared with single-center experiences previously documented.[21,22]

A systematic review, comparing open versus fenestrated versus antegrade parallel stent grafting, showed that regardless of the approach, cumulative 30-day mortality was 3.4%, 2.4%, and 5.3 respectively. Impaired renal function was noted in 18.5%, 9.8%, and 12% following open surgery, fenestrated endovascular aortic aneurysm repairs (F-EVAR), and Chimney-EVAR, respectively. Postoperative cardiac complications were noted in 11.3%, 3.7%, and 7.4%,

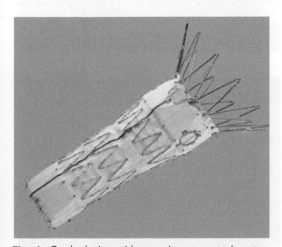

Fig. 1. Cook device with superior mesenteric artery scallop and fenestration. (Cook Medical, Bloomington, IN.)

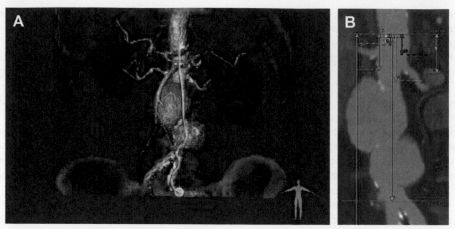

Fig. 2. (A) Yellow line indicates center line position throughout aorta and aneurysm sac. (B) Straightened image with measurements to visceral vessels and various points of interest for graft construction.

respectively (open vs F-EVAR: P<.001). The incidence of ischemic stroke was 0.1% and 0.3% following open surgery and F-EVAR, but 3.2% after Ch-EVAR (open vs Ch-EVAR: P = .002; F-EVAR vs Ch-EVAR: P = .012). Comparing the fenestrated approach directly to parallel stenting, intraoperative target vessel preservation

was 98.6% and 98.0%, respectively. A significant difference was found when assessing proximal type I endoleaks. They were found to be lower in the F-EVAR group compared with the Ch-EVAR (4.3% vs 10%, respectively, P = .002).[23]

Another approach to aortic side branches is to have grafts that are placed into the side

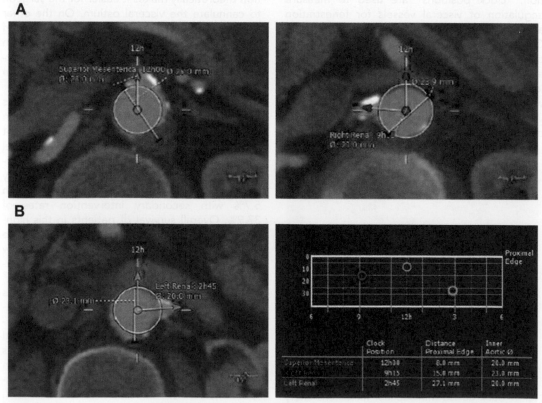

Fig. 3. (A) Clock positions of superior mesenteric artery at 1200 and right renal artery at 0915. (B) Clock position of left renal artery as shown above at 0245, and example of completed fenestration diagram for target vessels.

branches presewed onto the main body so that when deployed, the side branch stent is not a separate component of the graft but directly connected. These so-called branched endografts are also applicable to the arch vessels. These branches also typically come pre-cannulated within the sheath for ease with delivery.

A more recent technology, widely used in Europe but not yet FDA approved, looks to attack the aneurysm sac as well as create a flow lumen to bypass the aneurysm is termed Nellix. The Nellix system attempts to seal the aneurysm sac to limit the necessary secondary interventions as well as fixate the graft at the desired level with minimal neck length. It also uses a dual-lumen design to seal iliac distally regardless of diameter.[24] Nellix uses a polyethylene glycol–based polymer, which is injected in liquid form as a 2-part solution that cures in under 10 minutes at normal body temperature. This polymer is supposed to form a tight cross-linked polymer assembly that forms a density similar to that of blood and fills the aneurysm sac while maintaining light pressure on the aneurysm wall to prevent endoleaks.[25]

TROUBLESHOOTING/COMPLICATIONS

With any procedure, complications exist, and EVAR is no exception. The most common complication is an endoleak. Endoleaks are defined as a leak into the aneurysm sac after endovascular exclusion of the aneurysm.[26] It is associated with continued risk of aneurysm rupture. Five types of endoleaks exist and can been seen in **Fig. 4**. The most common type is type II, and these can be monitored through imaging surveillance. If associated with aneurysm growth, intervention is the typical recommendation, and they can most always be approached in an endovascular fashion. All type I and type III endoleaks found during the index procedure require intervention before leaving the operating room, and most found on follow-up require a procedure or vigilant monitoring. The reason that type I and III endoleaks carry such a strict recommendation is that they are the 2 endoleaks that most expose the aneurysm sac to systemic pressure, negating the purpose of the original procedure.[27]

Other complications associated with endovascular aneurysm repair include access site

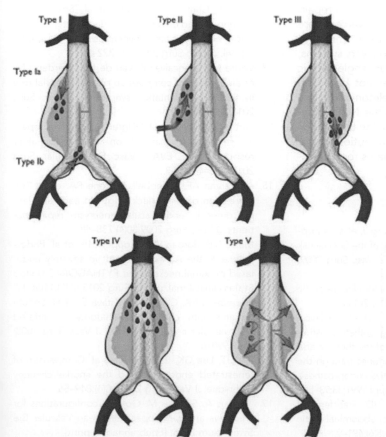

Fig. 4. Classification of endoleaks. Type Ia: leak at proximal graft fixation. Type Ib: leak at distal graft fixation. Type II: leak filling aneurysm sac retrograde from branch vessels (Inferior mesenteric artery, lumbar). Type III: leak through mechanical graft defect or junctional separation of components. Type IV: leak through graft fabric from porosity. Type V: So-called endotension because of continued sac growth with no identifiable source. (*From* Erbel R, Aboyans V, Boileau C, et al. 2014 ESC Guidelines on the diagnosis and treatment of aortic diseases. Eur Heart J 2014;35(41):2886. Available at: http://eurheartj.oxfordjournals. org/content/ehj/early/2014/08/28/ eurheartj.ehu281.full.pdf; with permission.)

complications, graft occlusion, graft infection, ischemic complications, contrast-dye–related complications, abdominal compartment syndrome, and postimplantation syndrome. These complications have been well documented in the literature and should be on the mind of every practitioner who deploys an aortic stent graft.

To that end, Aburahma and colleagues[28] describe a specific follow-up protocol for such cases to ensure absence of endoleaks as well as maintain perfusion to all stent grafts. All patients were encouraged to participate in postoperative surveillance protocol, which included computed tomographic angiography or color digital ultrasound imaging, or both, and plain abdominal radiography at 1, 6, and 12 months, and then every 12 months thereafter.

SUMMARY

Endovascular treatment of aortic abnormality is an excellent alternative option for patients who are not good candidates for conventional open surgery. Current research and design of newer endografts are concentrated on allowing for more widespread use of aortic endografts. These innovations attempt to push pass the original limitations of endovascular aneurysm repair. The most important limitations to overcome are achieving high-quality aortic neck "healthy" landing zone, smaller-diameter delivery systems, and endografts that allow for more angled aortic necks. In addition, technologies not based on the original design of metal skeleton and fabric overlay are emerging, such as the Nellix polymer. No matter the graft chosen, the technology allows for an excellent alternative option for patients who are not good candidates for conventional open surgery.

REFERENCES

1. Larsson E, Granath F, Swedenborg J, et al. A population-based case-control study of the familial risk of abdominal aortic aneurysm. J Vasc Surg 2009; 49(1):47–50.
2. Campbell WB. Mortality statistics for elective aortic aneurysms. Eur J Vasc Surg 1991;5(2):111–3.
3. Volodos NL, Karpovich IP, Troyan VI, et al. Clinical experience of the use of self-fixing synthetic prostheses for remote endoprosthetics of the thoracic and the abdominal aorta and iliac arteries through the femoral artery and as intraoperative endoprosthesis for aorta reconstruction. Vasa Suppl 1991;33:93–5.
4. Parodi JC, Palmaz JC, Barone HD. Transfemoral intraluminal graft implantation for abdominal aortic aneurysms. Ann Vasc Surg 1991;5(6):491–9.
5. Chuter TA, Donayre C, Wendt G. Bifurcated stent-grafts for endovascular repair of abdominal aortic aneurysm. Preliminary case reports. Surg Endosc 1994;8(7):800–2.
6. White GH, Yu W, May J, et al. A new nonstented balloon-expandable graft for straight or bifurcated endoluminal bypass. J Endovasc Surg 1994;1:16–24.
7. Kolvenbach R, Pinter L, Cagiannos C, et al. Remodeling of the aortic neck with a balloon-expandable stent graft in patients with complicated neck morphology. Vascular 2008;16(4):183–8.
8. Mehta M, Valdes FE, Nolte T, et al. One-year outcomes from an international study of the Ovation Abdominal Stent Graft system for endovascular aneurysm repair. J Vasc Surg 2014;59(1): 65–73.e1–3.
9. Fischer A, Wieneke H, Brauer H, et al. Metallic biomaterials for coronary stents. Z Kardiol 2001;90(4): 251–62.
10. Thierry B, Merhi Y, Bilodeau L, et al. Nitinol versus stainless steel stents: acute thrombogenicity study in an ex vivo porcine model. Biomaterials 2002; 23(14):2997–3005.
11. Stoeckel D, Pelton A, Duerig T. Self-expanding nitinol stents: material and design considerations. Eur Radiol 2004;14(2):292–301.
12. Lin PH, Chen C, Bush RL, et al. Small-caliber heparin-coated ePTFE grafts reduce platelet deposition and neointimal hyperplasia in a baboon model. J Vasc Surg 2004;39:1322–8.
13. Voute MT, Goncalves B, van de Luijtgaarden KM, et al. Stent graft composition plays a material role in the postimplantation syndrome. J Vasc Surg 2012;56(6):1503–9.
14. Sartipy F, Lindstrom D, Gillgren P, et al. The impact of stent graft material on the inflammatory response after EVAR. Vasc Endovascular Surg 2015;49(3–4):79–83.
15. Aburahma AF, Campbell J, Stone PA, et al. The correlation of aortic neck length to early and late outcomes in endovascular aneurysm repair patients. J Vasc Surg 2009;50(4):738–48.
16. Malas MB, Jordan WD, Cooper MA, et al. Performance of the Aorfix endograft in severely angulated proximal necks in the PYTHAGORAS United States clinical trial. J Vasc Surg 2015;62(5):1108–17.
17. Greenberg RK, Clair D, Srivastava S, et al. Should patients with challenging anatomy be offered endovascular aneurysm repair? J Vasc Surg 2003; 38(5):990–6.
18. Lee JT, Lee GK, Chandra V, et al. Comparison of fenestrated endografts and the snorkel/chimney technique. J Vasc Surg 2014;60(4):849–56.
19. Tanious A, Shames M. Optimal configurations for chimneys and periscopes. European Vascular Bio Symposium 2015. [Epub ahead of print].

20. Lee JT, Donas KP, Torsello G, et al. Collected world experience of the snorkel/chimney endovascular technique in the treatment of complex aortic aneurysms: the PERICLES registry. Ann Surg 2015;262(3): 546–53 [discussion: 552–3].

21. Scali ST, Feezor RJ, Chang CK, et al. Critical analysis of results after chimney endovascular aortic aneurysm repair raises cause for concern. J Vasc Surg 2014;60(4):865–74.

22. Patel RP, Katsargyris A, Verhoeven ELG, et al. Endovascular aortic aneurysm repair with chimney and snorkel grafts: indications, techniques and results. Cardiovasc Intervent Radiol 2013; 36(6):1443–51.

23. Katsargyris A, Oikonomou K, Klonaris C, et al. Comparison of outcomes with open, fenestrated, and chimney graft repair of juxtarenal aneurysms: are we ready for a paradigm shift? J Endovasc Ther 2013;20(2):159–69.

24. Krievins DK, Holden A, Savlovskis J, et al. EVAR using the Nellix sac-anchoring endoprosthesis: treatment of favourable and adverse anatomy. Eur J Vasc Endovasc Surg 2011;42(1):38–46.

25. Nellix endovascular aneurysm sealing system. Endologix, Inc; 2016. Available at: http://www.endologix.com/products/nellix/nellix.php. Accessed January 12, 2016.

26. Chaikof EL, Blankensteijn JD, Harris PL, et al. Reporting standards for endovascular aortic aneurysm repair. J Vasc Surg 2002;35(5):1048–60.

27. Veith FJ, Baum RA, Ohki T, et al. Nature and significance of endoleaks and endotension: summary of opinions expressed at an international conference. J Vasc Surg 2002;35(5):1029–35.

28. Aburahma AF, Campbell JE, Mousa AY, et al. Clinical outcomes for hostile versus favorable aortic neck anatomy in endovascular aortic aneurysm repair using modular devices. J Vasc Surg 2011;54(1):13–21.

Pathology of Endovascular Stents

Kenta Nakamura, MD[a,b,c,]*, John H. Keating, DVM[d],
Elazer Reuven Edelman, MD, PhD[b,e]

KEYWORDS

- Coronary artery disease • Pathology • Bare metal stent • Drug-eluting stent • In-stent restenosis
- In-stent thrombosis • Atherosclerosis • Neoatherosclerosis

KEY POINTS

- Improvement in endovascular stent performance has occurred iteratively over decades and highlights the ability to optimize physiologic function and minimize pathologic response through design.
- Pathology associated with endovascular stents most commonly manifests clinically as progressive angina due to in-stent restenosis (ISR) or acute myocardial infarction (MI) due to in-stent thrombosis (IST).
- ISR is mediated by neointima hyperplasia due to a complex interaction of biological, mechanical, technical, and patient-specific factors.
- Delayed arterial healing and possibly incomplete stent coverage by endothelium predominantly mediate IST, leading to plaque fissuring and rupture.
- Neoatherosclerosis develops over months to years as opposed to decades with native coronary atherosclerosis and contributes to late and very late IST (VLST).

INTRODUCTION

Coronary artery disease (CAD) represents the leading cause of death worldwide, attributed to more than 17.5 million deaths annually, accounting for approximately 1 of every 3 deaths.[1] In the United States, contemporary decreases in CAD-related mortality correlate with the 2 decades after the Surgeon General report on the ills of tobacco, the Framingham Heart Study identification of cardiac risk factors with lifestyle modification, and the widespread acceptance and accessibility of evidence-based use of percutaneous coronary intervention (PCI).[2] The technologies underpinning PCI have evolved iteratively from balloon angioplasty to increasingly advanced metallic stent platforms with various drug chemistries to self-degrading nonmetallic scaffolds. Large-scale clinical trials have validated the safety and efficacy of successive generations of stents. Equally important preclinical[3–5] and pathology studies provide complementary insight to reconcile adverse events; refine clinical protocols, such as optimal use of antithrombotic therapy; and drive innovation for development of next-generation stents.

NATIVE CORONARY ARTERY DISEASE

The fundamental pathogenesis of native coronary atherosclerosis has been described for decades but only recently have the specific

Financial Disclosure: Nothing to disclose for all authors.
Funding: This article was supported in part by the National Institutes of Health (R01 GM-49039) to Dr E.R. Edelman.
[a] CBSET, Applied Sciences, 500 Shire Way, Lexington, MA 02421, USA; [b] Institute for Medical Engineering and Science, Massachusetts Institute of Technology, 77 Massachusetts Avenue, Building E25-438, Cambridge, MA 02139, USA; [c] Division of Cardiology, Department of Medicine, Massachusetts General Hospital, Harvard Medical School, 55 Fruit Street, Yawkey 5B, Boston, MA 02114, USA; [d] CBSET, Pathology, 500 Shire Way, Lexington, MA 02421, USA; [e] Division of Cardiovascular Medicine, Department of Medicine, Brigham and Women's Hospital, Harvard Medical School, 75 Francis Street, Boston, MA 02115, USA
* Corresponding author. 55 Fruit Street, Yawkey 5B, Boston, MA 02114.
E-mail address: knakamura@cbset.org

nuances of these processes been characterized, particularly with respect to coronary intervention. As early as the 1970s, the importance of arterial injury in the establishment of atherosclerosis was recognized in the context of vascular smooth muscle cell activation and proliferation.[6,7] The injury model shifted toward a more complex understanding underpinned by inflammation and integration of recognized cardiac risk factors, such as hyperlipidemia, hypertension, diabetes, and smoking.[8,9] The pathogenesis of atherosclerosis as a chronic inflammatory disease marked by progressive vascular wall injury became further defined and synchronized with clinical events, such as plaque rupture and acute thrombosis comprising the acute coronary syndrome.[10–13] Establishment and maturation of atherosclerotic plaque is now well recognized as a progression from deposition and subsequent oxidation of free cholesterol, intimal thickening, and xanthoma (fatty streak) development to infiltration and lipid-avid macrophages, formation of a necrotic core, and progression to fibroatheroma predisposed to rupture and thrombosis.[14,15] Introduction of routine PCI transformed the management of CAD and provided serial clinical data that emphasized the nonlinear nature of atherosclerotic plaque development: luminal stenosis alone is not a predictor of future clinical events[16] and bore the concept of the "vulnerable plaque."[17] Not all plaques are created equal and some are more prone to rupture than others. Contemporary understanding of atherosclerosis now classifies the vulnerable plaque as thin-cap fibroatheroma (TCFA), predisposed to acute plaque rupture, and incorporates other pathologic mechanisms of thrombosis, such as healed plaque rupture, surface erosion, and calcified nodules.[13] Antemortem identification of such rupture-prone plaques has yet to be realized, frustrating current clinical management paradigms and causing some investigators to question the very existence of such lesions.

PATHOLOGY OF BALLOON ANGIOPLASTY

The introduction of PCI with balloon angioplasty marked the first widely adopted technique to directly alter the natural history of atherosclerosis. Angioplasty alone, however, proved a temporizing therapy, owing to the traumatic and inconsistent nature of plaque modification.[18–20] Although initially perceived and perhaps hoped to result in permanent deformation, the end result was far more elastic, with reversible displacement that more often recoiled

back to its original dimension. Associated tissue damage was, however, real and injury to endothelium, intima, and media promoted rapid restenosis within weeks to months of therapy in addition to further precipitating the acute complications of arterial dissection and recoil.[21,22] The specific effects of balloon angioplasty on the arterial wall have been defined serially: vascular recoil and contraction after balloon dilation; injury to the intima and dissection of the media; and inflammatory activation and proliferation of vascular smooth muscle cells, resulting in rapid neointimal hyperplasia, extracellular matrix deposition, and negative vascular remodeling.[23–26] To combat the loss of effect and minimize the extent of injury, PCI incorporated the use of permanent metal mesh implants—bare metal stents (BMSs)—after balloon angioplasty to rigidly support the arterial lumen, control arterial dissection, and prevent acute arterial recoil to good effect.[22,27] Stent placement, nevertheless, necessarily modifies the stenotic lesion and alters arterial architecture, inducing arterial injury not unlike balloon angioplasty.

PATHOLOGY OF BARE METAL STENTS

BMS deployment typically results in neointimal hyperplasia, which is driven by vascular smooth muscle cell proliferation and associated with macrophage accumulation and neovascularization. Neointimal hyperplasia may be distributed either along the length of the stent or focally.[24,28–34] During the first 2 weeks of BMS placement, fibrin, platelets, and acute inflammatory cells are localized to the stent struts, in particular those embedded within the necrotic plaque core or injured arterial wall media (Figs. 1 and 2).[35,36] In the weeks and months that follow, neointimal hyperplasia and then, increasingly, extracellular matrix deposition contribute to neointimal growth.[37] In association with a metallic scaffold, the arterial architecture is altered such that homeostatic expansive remodeling occurs (the so-called Glagov phenomenon[38]) and physiologic vasodilation is impaired. Incremental plaque development thus directly impinges on lumen area, rapidly precipitating ISR at an accelerated rate compared with native disease. Through these mechanisms, ISR accelerates early and seems to peak at approximately 6 months and, in its ultimate state, may precipitate recrudescence of clinical symptoms requiring repeat target lesions revascularization (TLR). By the first year after BMS placement, however, the neointima generally stabilizes and luminal diameter

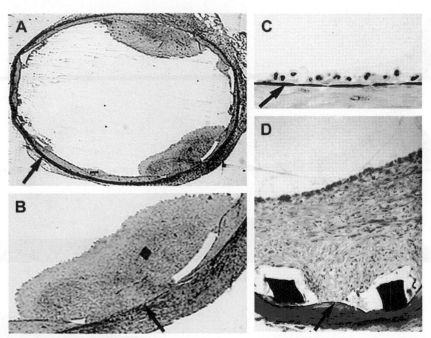

Fig. 1. (A) Acute thrombosis and subacute thrombosis observed after endovascular BMS placement. (B) Is a zoomed in lower right corner of *panel A*. (C) Three days after endovascular BMS placement (Verhoeff elastic tissue stain), adherent mononuclear cells line the internal elastic lamina (*arrow*). (D) Two weeks after BMS placement (modified Russell-Movat pentachrome stain), robust neointimal hyperplasia is observed separating the lumen from the internal elastic lamina (*arrows*). Stent struts (*black rectangles*); postprocessing effect (*white area*). Internal elastic lamina (*Black Arrow*). (*Adapted from* Rogers C, Parikh S, Seifert P, et al. Endogenous cell seeding. Remnant endothelium after stenting enhances vascular repair. Circulation 1996;94(11):2912; with permission.)

may regress.[39,40] The authors' laboratory reported the importance of the geometric configuration of stent struts in addition to surface material in predicting the degree of arterial injury and inflammation (Fig. 3).[5] This idea not only led to introduction of a range of stent designs but also suggested that drugs might best have their effects if delivered in the vicinity of the implanted devices and, to this end, drug-eluting stents (DESs) engineered with advanced materials and antiproliferative properties were developed to prevent short-term vascular injury, neointimal hyperplasia, and thrombosis.

PATHOLOGY OF DRUG-ELUTING STENTS: IN-STENT RESTENOSIS

DESs are defined by an elutable drug delivered to the arterial wall via controlled release from a polymer matrix that uniformly coats the metallic stent. First-generation DESs used either the cytostatic agent sirolimus to suppress smooth muscle cell activation by arresting the G_1 phase of the cell cycle or the cytotoxic agent paclitaxel to interfere with microtubular depolymerization.[41] Introduction of DESs significantly

reduced ISR and TLR in several pivotal randomized clinical trials.[42–45] It was still the case that lesion complexity drove ISR.[46,47] Likely mechanisms to explain ISR with DESs were organized into 4 primary domains: (1) biological factors, including vascular injury,[33] malapposition,[48] and nonuniform drug delivery[49–51]; (2) mechanical factors, including stent underexpansion,[52,53] hemodynamic stress, and stent fracture[54,55]; (3) technical factors, including barotrauma,[43] stent gap and overlap,[56] and residual untreated plaque[57]; and (4) patient-specific factors, such as comorbidities,[58] drug resistance,[59,60] and hypersensitivity[61,62] (Fig. 4). Detailed pathologic study of stents revealed direct injury to the media or lipid-rich necrotic core of plaques by penetrating stent struts, thus predisposing to ISR.[33,63] Unique pathologic responses are observed between stent composition, consistent with expected differences in drug biology.[64] For example, response to sirolimus stents is often characterized by malapposition due to robust inflammation and intimal infiltration of eosinophils, lymphocytes, and giant cells whereas response to paclitaxel-eluting stents included malapposition induced by excessive parastrut

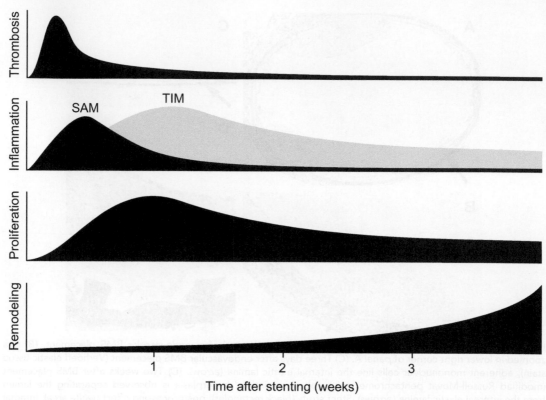

Fig. 2. Activity of the 4 primary components of arterial injury after stent placement. Platelet-rich thrombosis peaks 3 to 4 days after stent deployment especially over areas of strut injury. Concomitant inflammation is initially mediated by surface-adherent monocytes (SAM) recruited to the injury site that then migrate into the neointima as tissue-infiltrating monocytes (TIM) and accumulate around the stent struts as giant cells. Vascular smooth muscle cell proliferation peaks 7 days after stent deployment coincident with the transition of SAM to TIM and continues for weeks afterward. Extracellular matrix deposition in the adventitia, tunica media, and neointima accelerates at week 3 after stent deployment and underlies arterial remodeling and subsequent luminal narrowing. (*Adapted from* Edelman ER, Rogers C. Pathobiologic responses to stenting. Am J Cardiol 1998;81(7A):6E; with permission.)

fibrin deposition.[65] These processes ultimately invoke the common pathologic response of neo-intimal hyperplasia and inflammation, leading to extracellular matrix deposition and negative vascular remodeling.

NEOATHEROSCLEROSIS

Contemporary long-term pathologic studies have identified a novel mechanism of in-stent atherosclerosis, which is independent of native atherosclerosis and develops rapidly within the neointima. This is so-called neoatherosclerosis, an important mediator of ISR with DESs.[66–68] Neoatherosclerosis is characterized by accelerated plaque progression in which there is accumulation of peristrut macrophage, and lipid-rich foam cells, which organize as fibroatheroma on the luminal surface and deeper within the neointima.[67] Neoatherosclerosis

predisposes to plaque fissure and rupture that may present symptomatically as acute, often catastrophic, thrombosis or may be clinically silent, forming substrate for ISR and chronic thrombotic occlusion.[68] Compared with BMSs, DESs are associated with neointima with more abundant proteoglycan in the extracellular matrix, which is highly avid to lipoproteins.[69,70] Local disruption of laminar blood flow by stent struts induces alterations in shear stress that stimulates endothelium to express the intercellular adhesion molecule 1 and vascular cell adhesion protein [or molecule] 1, allowing transmigration of circulating monocytes into the neointima where they activate into macrophages, load with lipid, and form foam cells.[71–73] The disrupted fluid dynamics also promote platelet and fibrin deposition[67] and predispose to thrombus formation. Over time, a necrotic core of free cholesterol devoid of extracellular

No coating   Polymer coating

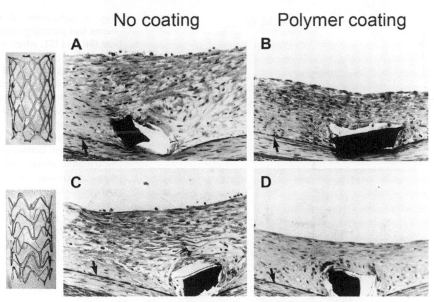

Fig. 3. Stent surface and geometry significantly affect vascular injury and neointimal hyperplasia. Two BMSs where fabricated using the same metal, process, and net surface area, on in a slotted tube (*upper left panel*) and the other corrugated ring (*lower left panel*) configuration and implanted in rabbit femoral arteries. Histologic examination was performed on methyl methacylate–embedded specimens harvested 2 weeks after placement. (*A, B*) Uncoated surface; (*C, D*) polymer-coated surface. Internal elastic lamina (*arrow*), stent struts (*black rectangles*), and (*C, D*) polymer material (*white rim circumscribing stent strut*). (*Adapted from* Rogers C, Edelman ER. Endovascular stent design dictates experimental restenosis and thrombosis. Circulation 1995;91(12):2996 and 2999; with permission.)

matrix and sometimes exhibiting calcification forms within the neoatherosclerotic plaque from direct apoptosis of foam cells and smooth muscle cells.[74–76] Unlike native atherosclerosis, pathologic neointimal thickening does not occur within the stented neoatherosclerotic plaques, and lesions progress rapidly with superficial necrotic cores that are inherently less stable and progress more rapidly into late fibroatheromas.[68] Moreover, unlike intimal xanthomas, or fatty streaks, in native atherosclerosis, which may remain stable or regress,[77,78] neoatherosclerosis lesions invariably progress to necrotic cores though apoptosis.[13] Intramural hemorrhage from fissuring of the luminal surface or leaking of the adventitial vasa vasorum further destabilizes the neoatherosclerotic plaque.[79] The fibrous cap eventually thins, forming vulnerable plaque, or TCFA, at high-risk for plaque rupture[67] and a histologic predictor of future coronary event.[13]

The precise mechanism of neoatherosclerosis remains unclear, but dysfunctional endothelial barrier function due to incompetent or incomplete endothelial coverage of the stent is thought to play a key role.[79,80] This is supported by clinical evidence that neoatherosclerosis develops more rapidly with DESs than BMSs.[65] Mechanical injury by stent struts denudes the

arterial wall of endothelium. The antiproliferative effects of DESs prevent maturation of the regenerating endothelium, further impairing endothelial integrity. This may explain the more pronounced and rapid development of neoatherosclerosis in DESs than in BMSs.[65,81] Specifically, poorly functional endothelium is characterized by reduced intercellular junctions, antithrombin expression, and nitric oxide production, which are observed more commonly in DESs compared with BMSs.[71,80] The antiproliferative effects of drug and delayed endothelial healing are further compounded when stent struts violate the necrotic core where drug clearance and repair mechanisms are reduced in the avascular space.[67] Classically, circulating monocytes infiltrate the intima through the damaged endothelium and differentiate into macrophages, which load with lipid and undergo apoptosis, leaving xanthomas.[67,80] More recently, direct transdifferentiation of smooth muscle cells into macrophages has been described, using elegant in vitro lineage tracing experiments of native atherosclerosis.[82] Whether a similar process of phenotype transition occurs in neoatherosclerosis is unknown. Neoatherosclerosis may result in ISR or more often serves as substrate for plaque instability and eventual rupture and thrombosis.

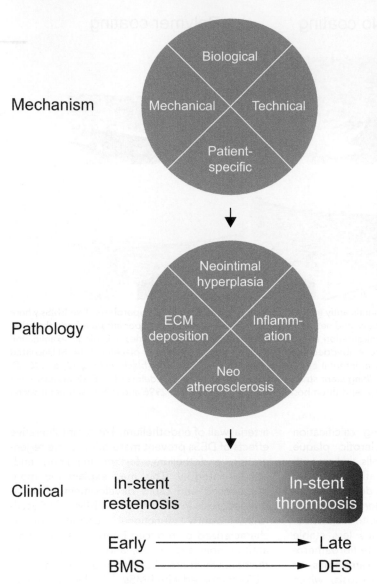

Mechanism

Pathology

Clinical

Fig. 4. Schematic of the mechanisms and pathology mediating clinical ISR and IST, which likely lie on a shared continuum that shifts from early events associated with BMSs to late events, associated with DESs. Biological factors include vascular injury, malapposition with fibrin deposition, and nonuniform drug delivery; mechanical factors include stent underexpansion, hemodynamic stress, and stent fracture; technical factors include balloon barotrauma, stent gap and overlap, and residual untreated plaque; and patient-specific factors include comorbidities, drug resistance, and hypersensitivity. ECM, extracellular matrix.

PATHOLOGY OF DRUG-ELUTING STENTS: LATE IN-STENT THROMBOSIS

A complementary pathologic process to ISR is IST[83,84] (see Fig. 4). Whereas ISR is a progressive process often leading to stable angina and rarely (approximately 10%), MI, IST is a catastrophic cause of acute MI and sudden death[84] and may present as late stent failure.[58,85–87] The biological, mechanical, technical, and patient-specific factors described for ISR also contribute to a lesser extent to IST.[65,79,88,89] Neoatherosclerosis has more recently been studied as a significant substrate for late-stent thrombosis (LST)/VLST in both BMSs and DESs. Late stent failure

has been ascribed to neoatherosclerosis in numerous pathology and intracoronary imaging studies.[66,90,91] Although DESs successfully forestall early development of ISR through inhibition of intimal hyperplasia, delayed healing of the stented region also predisposes to the complication of late IST.[79,85,88,92–95] Although initial studies reported comparable rates of IST with DESs compared with BMSs within the first 6 to 12 months of stenting,[96–98] late thrombosis became recognized with longer follow-up.[99] The benefit of decreased ISR with DESs was thus partially counterbalanced by increased risk of IST. Long-term rates of MI and death beyond 1 year after stenting were not significantly different between first-generation DESs and BMSs.[99] In addition to acute and subacute IST within 1 month of stenting, LST occurring 30 days to 1 year and VLST occurring after 1 year are well-recognized complications of first-generation DESs.[92] The primary substrate for LST/VLST in DESs is delayed arterial healing and possibly inadequate stent coverage and incorporation into the vessel wall.[80,88,93,100] The ratio of uncovered to total stent area as determined by histology is a significant predictor of LST.[93] Thrombosis by plaque rupture may be mediated by lesions in the vicinity of thrombus initiation, likely either within the stented region or in the immediate vicinity. Intracoronary imaging studies suggest that plaque rupture occurs more frequently at the nonstented region immediately adjacent to the stent edge, causing thrombosis of the stented region.[101,102] Autopsy studies, however, show neoatherosclerosis originating within and restricted to stented regions, suggesting flow disturbances at the native-stent transition may play a role in stented plaque rupture and thrombosis.[67]

SECOND-GENERATION DRUG-ELUTING STENTS

Second-generation DES technology provided improvements in drug, polymer, and metal properties together with lower-profile geometries that address many of the biological, mechanical, and technical factors that underlie first-generation DES failure. Nevertheless, second-generation DESs remain vulnerable to long-term stent failure. The second-generation cobalt-chromium everolimus-eluting stent (CoCr-EES) has been consistently superior to first-generation DESs with reduction in ISR and TRL, MI, and cardiac death in high-quality randomized control trials.[94,103–107] Second-generation DES technology has ameliorated the risk of ISR with improved arterial healing and reduced the risk of IST,[108–110] yet stent failure remains a known complication and cumulative incidence of ISR and TLR increases with all generations of DES platforms over time.[86,111–113] It is suggested that in total, all of the design improvements that accompany CoCr-EES enhance healing or reduce initial injury with greater endothelial regeneration[114] and less inflammation and fibrin deposition compared with sirolimus and paclitaxel-eluting first-generation DESs.[115] Evidence for neoatherosclerosis was noted for CoCr-EES at 270 days, much later than first-generation siroliumus-DESs and paclitaxel-DESs, in which neoatherosclerosis was observed at 120 days and 70 days,

respectively.[115] The more gradual development of neoatherosclerosis in second-generation versus first-generation DESs may promote more stable lesion development, because high-risk features like TCFA and plaque rupture were not observed with second-generation DESs.[116] Although second-generation DESs seem to promote greater endothelial healing and more stable neoatherosclerosis, the overall incidence of neoatherosclerosis, however, is similar across DES generations,[110,115,117] and thrombosis risk remains a concern clinically.[111] Second-generation DESs are increasingly acknowledged to have a catch-up phenomenon of neointimal growth that correlates with delayed arterial healing.[111,118]

Further improvements in PCI technology and techniques have enabled treatment of more complex disease, such as bifurcation lesions posing higher risk for complications. The pathology associated with DESs in bifurcation lesions is accentuated at the bifurcation carina, which is a high shear stress area where arterial healing is impaired compared with the lateral wall. This results in greater fibrin deposition, necrotic core accumulation, and plaque thickness at the carina compared with the lower shear stress lateral walls.[119] Efforts to improve stent material and architecture as well as polymer coating have been eclipsed by technology to mitigate or eliminate these components from next-generation devices.

NEXT-GENERATION STENTS AND SCAFFOLDS

Persistence of polymer coating in first-generation DESs after drug delivery is problematic as a stimulus of peristrut inflammation, delayed arterial healing, ISR, and IST. This has led to efforts to minimize polymer coating or develop polymer-free scaffolds.[80,120–122] The next iteration of the DES involves further refinement of drug and polymer matrix, including stents with asymmetric coatings, biodegradable polymer materials, or controlled drug delivery not requiring polymer coating. These DESs with novel polymer materials or drug delivery strategies are thought be transformed into BMSs after the acute and short-term benefit of drug elution is complete. The underlying hypothesis in support of the totally erodible materials is that long-term presence of a rigid metallic stent in the arterial environment inhibits physiologic vascular tone and vasomotion[123] and is a nidus for late complications like fracture, neoatherosclerosis, and LST/VLST. To this end, bioresorbable scaffolds (BRSs) that degrade after lesion pacification have been in development since the early conceptualization of endovascular stents with the pioneering Igaki-Tamai BRS (Igaki Medical Planning Company, Kyoto, Japan) and succeeded by several BRSs currently in clinical trial. The everolimus-eluting Absorb Bioresorbable Vascular Scaffold (BVS) (Abbott Vascular; Abbott Park, Illinois) and DESolve Novolimus Eluting Bioresorbable Coronary Scaffold (Elixir Medical Corporation; Sunnyvale, California) have received Conformité Européenne mark approval in 2011 and 2013, respectively, and await Food and Drug Administration approval.[124] Early experience with the Absorb BVS has been promising[125,126] but must be tempered by reports of increased rates of acute thrombosis.[127,128] Although BRSs seem to address the longer-term complications of delayed arterial healing and neoatherosclerosis by complete degradation, they may be subject to the complications encountered with early stent designs. Specifically, large and bulky strut architecture and propensity for underexpansion create local disruption of laminar flow and increased hemodynamic stress.[5,63,129] The inflammatory response to the Absorb BVS seems to peak at 1 month and largely abates by 3 months with positive expansile remodeling after 12 months in nonatherosclerotic swine but may persist for longer in humans.[130,131] Small cohorts of patients have demonstrated similar increases in lumen diameter in imaging studies.[132] The anticipated benefits of BRS technology, notably restoration of vascular tone and vasomotion and reduced risk of LST and VLST, require further clinical study. Human pathology and imaging studies will again provide important insights into the pathophysiology and performance of BRS technology.

SUMMARY

The generalized pathology associated with endovascular stents is characterized by acute arterial injury, neointimal hyperplasia and inflammation, extracellular matrix deposition, and negative vascular remodeling. Numerous biological, mechanical, and technical factors contribute to ISR and IST, and evolution of PCI technologies has led to an amazing array of studies defining this vascular pathobiology in a synergistic manner and addressed these pathologies, seeking to balance the acute, chronic, and long-term requirements for lesion pacification and vascular healing. Commercially available DESs are effective but limited by late and very late complications of IST, mediated principally

by incomplete endothelial healing as a consequence of the antiproliferative effects that oppose early ISR. Neoatherosclerosis is another mechanism increasingly recognized as a cause of LST and VLST. Next-generation DES and BRS platforms address the pathology observed with prior stent designs and will likely be complemented by adjunctive devices like drug-eluting balloons and specialized bifurcation designs. Careful attention to the pathophysiologic response to these new technologies, with rigorous preclinical, autopsy, and in vivo imaging studies, will inform continued advancements. Successful endovascular stent design will ultimately match the specific attributes of the stent with the expected pathology underlying the exact clinical setting, including integration of lesion-specific and patient-specific determinants of stent failure.

ACKNOWLEDGMENTS

The authors thank Dr Abraham R. Tzafriri for thoughtful discussion and editorial assistance.

REFERENCES

1. World Health Organization Global Status Report on Noncommunicable Diseases. 2014. Available at: http://apps.who.int/iris/bitstream/10665/148114/1/9789241564854_eng.pdf. Accessed December 20, 2015.
2. Mozaffarian D, Benjamin EJ, Go AS, et al. Heart disease and stroke statistics–2015 update: a report from the American Heart Association. Circulation 2015;131(4):e29–322.
3. Schwartz RS, Edelman ER, Carter A, et al. Drug-eluting stents in preclinical studies: recommended evaluation from a consensus group. Circulation 2002;106(14):1867–73.
4. Joner M, Byrne RA. The importance of preclinical research in contemporary interventional cardiology. EuroIntervention 2010;6(1):19–23.
5. Rogers C, Edelman ER. Endovascular stent design dictates experimental restenosis and thrombosis. Circulation 1995;91(12):2995–3001.
6. Ross R, Glomset JA. The pathogenesis of atherosclerosis (first of two parts). N Engl J Med 1976;295(7):369–77.
7. Ross R, Glomset JA. The pathogenesis of atherosclerosis (second of two parts). N Engl J Med 1976;295(8):420–5.
8. Hansson GK. Inflammation, atherosclerosis, and coronary artery disease. N Engl J Med 2005;352(16):1685–95.
9. Libby P. Inflammation in atherosclerosis. Nature 2002;420(6917):868–74.

10. Fuster V, Badimon L, Badimon JJ, et al. The pathogenesis of coronary artery disease and the acute coronary syndromes (1). N Engl J Med 1992; 326(4):242–50.

11. Fuster V, Badimon L, Badimon JJ, et al. The pathogenesis of coronary artery disease and the acute coronary syndromes (2). N Engl J Med 1992; 326(5):310–8.

12. Stary HC, Chandler AB, Dinsmore RE, et al. A definition of advanced types of atherosclerotic lesions and a histological classification of atherosclerosis. A report from the Committee on Vascular Lesions of the Council on Arteriosclerosis, American Heart Association. Circulation 1995;92(5):1355–74.

13. Virmani R, Kolodgie FD, Burke AP, et al. Lessons from sudden coronary death: a comprehensive morphological classification scheme for atherosclerotic lesions. Arterioscler Thromb Vasc Biol 2000;20(5):1262–75.

14. Davies MJ, Thomas A. Thrombosis and acute coronary-artery lesions in sudden cardiac ischemic death. N Engl J Med 1984;310(18):1137–40.

15. Falk E, Nakano M, Bentzon JF, et al. Update on acute coronary syndromes: the pathologists' view. Eur Heart J 2013;34(10):719–28.

16. Glaser R, Selzer F, Faxon DP, et al. Clinical progression of incidental, asymptomatic lesions discovered during culprit vessel coronary intervention. Circulation 2005;111(2):143–9.

17. Stary HC, Blankenhorn DH, Chandler AB, et al. A definition of the intima of human arteries and of its atherosclerosis-prone regions. A report from the Committee on Vascular Lesions of the Council on Arteriosclerosis, American Heart Association. Circulation 1992;85(1):391–405.

18. Dangas G, Fuster V. Management of restenosis after coronary intervention. Am Heart J 1996;132(2 Pt 1):428–36.

19. Ormiston JA, Stewart FM, Roche AH, et al. Late regression of the dilated site after coronary angioplasty: a 5-year quantitative angiographic study. Circulation 1997;96(2):468–74.

20. Dangas GD, Claessen BE, Caixeta A, et al. In-stent restenosis in the drug-eluting stent era. J Am Coll Cardiol 2010;56(23):1897–907.

21. Block PC, Myler RK, Stertzer S, et al. Morphology after transluminal angioplasty in human beings. N Engl J Med 1981;305(7):382–5.

22. Serruys PW, de Jaegere P, Kiemeneij F, et al. A comparison of balloon-expandable-stent implantation with balloon angioplasty in patients with coronary artery disease. Benestent Study Group. N Engl J Med 1994;331(8):489–95.

23. Libby P, Tanaka H. The molecular bases of restenosis. Prog Cardiovasc Dis 1997;40(2):97–106.

24. Lowe HC, Oesterle SN, Khachigian LM. Coronary in-stent restenosis: current status and future strategies. J Am Coll Cardiol 2002; 39(2):183–93.

25. Danenberg HD, Welt FG, Walker M 3rd, et al. Systemic inflammation induced by lipopolysaccharide increases neointimal formation after balloon and stent injury in rabbits. Circulation 2002; 105(24):2917–22.

26. Schoenhagen P, Ziada KM, Vince DG, et al. Arterial remodeling and coronary artery disease: the concept of "dilated" versus "obstructive" coronary atherosclerosis. J Am Coll Cardiol 2001; 38(2):297–306.

27. Fischman DL, Leon MB, Baim DS, et al. A randomized comparison of coronary-stent placement and balloon angioplasty in the treatment of coronary artery disease. Stent Restenosis Study Investigators. N Engl J Med 1994;331(8):496–501.

28. Hoffmann R, Mintz GS, Dussaillant GR, et al. Patterns and mechanisms of in-stent restenosis. A serial intravascular ultrasound study. Circulation 1996;94(6):1247–54.

29. Kearney M, Pieczek A, Haley L, et al. Histopathology of in-stent restenosis in patients with peripheral artery disease. Circulation 1997;95(8): 1998–2002.

30. Kornowski R, Hong MK, Tio FO, et al. In-stent restenosis: contributions of inflammatory responses and arterial injury to neointimal hyperplasia. J Am Coll Cardiol 1998;31(1):224–30.

31. Rogers C, Welt FG, Karnovsky MJ, et al. Monocyte recruitment and neointimal hyperplasia in rabbits. Coupled inhibitory effects of heparin. Arterioscler Thromb Vasc Biol 1996;16(10):1312–8.

32. Komatsu R, Ueda M, Naruko T, et al. Neointimal tissue response at sites of coronary stenting in humans: macroscopic, histological, and immunohistochemical analyses. Circulation 1998;98(3):224–33.

33. Farb A, Weber DK, Kolodgie FD, et al. Morphological predictors of restenosis after coronary stenting in humans. Circulation 2002;105(25): 2974–80.

34. Farb A, Kolodgie FD, Hwang JY, et al. Extracellular matrix changes in stented human coronary arteries. Circulation 2004;110(8):940–7.

35. Farb A, Sangiorgi G, Carter AJ, et al. Pathology of acute and chronic coronary stenting in humans. Circulation 1999;99(1):44–52.

36. Edelman ER, Rogers C. Pathobiologic responses to stenting. Am J Cardiol 1998;81(7A):4E–6E.

37. Chung IM, Gold HK, Schwartz SM, et al. Enhanced extracellular matrix accumulation in restenosis of coronary arteries after stent deployment. J Am Coll Cardiol 2002;40(12):2072–81.

38. Glagov S, Weisenberg E, Zarins CK, et al. Compensatory enlargement of human atherosclerotic coronary arteries. N Engl J Med 1987;316(22): 1371–5.

39. Kimura T, Yokoi H, Nakagawa Y, et al. Three-year follow-up after implantation of metallic coronary-artery stents. N Engl J Med 1996;334(9):561–6.

40. Kuroda N, Kobayashi Y, Nameki M, et al. Intimal hyperplasia regression from 6 to 12 months after stenting. Am J Cardiol 2002;89(7):869–72.

41. Costa MA, Simon DI. Molecular basis of restenosis and drug-eluting stents. Circulation 2005;111(17):2257–73.

42. Stone GW, Ellis SG, Cox DA, et al. A polymer-based, paclitaxel-eluting stent in patients with coronary artery disease. N Engl J Med 2004;350(3):221–31.

43. Moses JW, Leon MB, Popma JJ, et al. Sirolimus-eluting stents versus standard stents in patients with stenosis in a native coronary artery. N Engl J Med 2003;349(14):1315–23.

44. Stettler C, Wandel S, Allemann S, et al. Outcomes associated with drug-eluting and bare-metal stents: a collaborative network meta-analysis. Lancet 2007;370(9591):937–48.

45. Morice MC, Serruys PW, Sousa JE, et al. A randomized comparison of a sirolimus-eluting stent with a standard stent for coronary revascularization. N Engl J Med 2002;346(23):1773–80.

46. Windecker S, Serruys PW, Wandel S, et al. Biolimus-eluting stent with biodegradable polymer versus sirolimus-eluting stent with durable polymer for coronary revascularisation (LEADERS): a randomised non-inferiority trial. Lancet 2008;372(9644):1163–73.

47. Morice MC, Colombo A, Meier B, et al. Sirolimus-vs paclitaxel-eluting stents in de novo coronary artery lesions: the REALITY trial: a randomized controlled trial. JAMA 2006;295(8):895–904.

48. Cook S, Wenaweser P, Togni M, et al. Incomplete stent apposition and very late stent thrombosis after drug-eluting stent implantation. Circulation 2007;115(18):2426–34.

49. Balakrishnan B, Tzafriri AR, Seifert P, et al. Strut position, blood flow, and drug deposition: implications for single and overlapping drug-eluting stents. Circulation 2005;111(22):2958–65.

50. Hwang CW, Levin AD, Jonas M, et al. Thrombosis modulates arterial drug distribution for drug-eluting stents. Circulation 2005;111(13):1619–26.

51. Hwang CW, Wu D, Edelman ER. Physiological transport forces govern drug distribution for stent-based delivery. Circulation 2001;104(5):600–5.

52. de Jaegere P, Mudra H, Figulla H, et al. Intravascular ultrasound-guided optimized stent deployment. Immediate and 6 months clinical and angiographic results from the Multicenter Ultrasound Stenting in Coronaries Study (MUSIC Study). Eur Heart J 1998;19(8):1214–23.

53. Mintz GS. Features and parameters of drug-eluting stent deployment discoverable by intravascular ultrasound. Am J Cardiol 2007;100(8B):26M–35M.

54. Doi H, Maehara A, Mintz GS, et al. Classification and potential mechanisms of intravascular ultrasound patterns of stent fracture. Am J Cardiol 2009;103(6):818–23.

55. Scheinert D, Scheinert S, Sax J, et al. Prevalence and clinical impact of stent fractures after femoropopliteal stenting. J Am Coll Cardiol 2005;45(2):312–5.

56. Kereiakes DJ, Wang H, Popma JJ, et al. Periprocedural and late consequences of overlapping Cypher sirolimus-eluting stents: pooled analysis of five clinical trials. J Am Coll Cardiol 2006;48(1):21–31.

57. Costa MA, Angiolillo DJ, Tannenbaum M, et al. Impact of stent deployment procedural factors on long-term effectiveness and safety of sirolimus-eluting stents (final results of the multicenter prospective STLLR trial). Am J Cardiol 2008;101(12):1704–11.

58. Doyle B, Rihal CS, O'Sullivan CJ, et al. Outcomes of stent thrombosis and restenosis during extended follow-up of patients treated with bare-metal coronary stents. Circulation 2007;116(21):2391–8.

59. Yusuf RZ, Duan Z, Lamendola DE, et al. Paclitaxel resistance: molecular mechanisms and pharmacologic manipulation. Curr Cancer Drug Targets 2003;3(1):1–19.

60. Huang S, Houghton PJ. Mechanisms of resistance to rapamycins. Drug Resist Updat 2001;4(6):378–91.

61. Koster R, Vieluf D, Kiehn M, et al. Nickel and molybdenum contact allergies in patients with coronary in-stent restenosis. Lancet 2000;356(9245):1895–7.

62. Nebeker JR, Virmani R, Bennett CL, et al. Hypersensitivity cases associated with drug-eluting coronary stents: a review of available cases from the Research on Adverse Drug Events and Reports (RADAR) project. J Am Coll Cardiol 2006;47(1):175–81.

63. Kolandaivelu K, Swaminathan R, Gibson WJ, et al. Stent thrombogenicity early in high-risk interventional settings is driven by stent design and deployment and protected by polymer-drug coatings. Circulation 2011;123(13):1400–9.

64. Levin AD, Vukmirovic N, Hwang CW, et al. Specific binding to intracellular proteins determines arterial transport properties for rapamycin and paclitaxel. Proc Natl Acad Sci U S A 2004;101(25):9463–7.

65. Nakazawa G, Finn AV, Vorpahl M, et al. Coronary responses and differential mechanisms of late stent thrombosis attributed to first-generation sirolimus- and paclitaxel-eluting stents. J Am Coll Cardiol 2011;57(4):390–8.

66. Kang SJ, Mintz GS, Akasaka T, et al. Optical coherence tomographic analysis of in-stent neoatherosclerosis after drug-eluting stent implantation. Circulation 2011;123(25):2954–63.

67. Otsuka F, Byrne RA, Yahagi K, et al. Neoatherosclerosis: overview of histopathologic findings and implications for intravascular imaging assessment. Eur Heart J 2015;36(32):2147–59.

68. Otsuka F, Joner M, Prati F, et al. Clinical classification of plaque morphology in coronary disease. Nat Rev Cardiol 2014;11(7):379–89.

69. Nakano M, Otsuka F, Yahagi K, et al. Human autopsy study of drug-eluting stents restenosis: histomorphological predictors and neointimal characteristics. Eur Heart J 2013;34(42):3304–13.

70. Williams KJ, Tabas I. The response-to-retention hypothesis of early atherogenesis. Arterioscler Thromb Vasc Biol 1995;15(5):551–61.

71. Otsuka F, Finn AV, Yazdani SK, et al. The importance of the endothelium in atherothrombosis and coronary stenting. Nat Rev Cardiol 2012;9(8): 439–53.

72. Jimenez JM, Davies PF. Hemodynamically driven stent strut design. Ann Biomed Eng 2009;37(8): 1483–94.

73. Davies PF. Hemodynamic shear stress and the endothelium in cardiovascular pathophysiology. Nat Clin Pract Cardiovasc Med 2009;6(1):16–26.

74. Tabas I. Consequences and therapeutic implications of macrophage apoptosis in atherosclerosis: the importance of lesion stage and phagocytic efficiency. Arterioscler Thromb Vasc Biol 2005; 25(11):2255–64.

75. Tulenko TN, Chen M, Mason PE, et al. Physical effects of cholesterol on arterial smooth muscle membranes: evidence of immiscible cholesterol domains and alterations in bilayer width during atherogenesis. J Lipid Res 1998;39(5):947–56.

76. Thorp E, Tabas I. Mechanisms and consequences of efferocytosis in advanced atherosclerosis. J Leukoc Biol 2009;86(5):1089–95.

77. Aikawa M, Rabkin E, Okada Y, et al. Lipid lowering by diet reduces matrix metalloproteinase activity and increases collagen content of rabbit atheroma: a potential mechanism of lesion stabilization. Circulation 1998;97(24):2433–44.

78. McGill HC Jr, McMahan CA, Herderick EE, et al. Effects of coronary heart disease risk factors on atherosclerosis of selected regions of the aorta and right coronary artery. PDAY Research Group. Pathobiological Determinants of Atherosclerosis in Youth. Arterioscler Thromb Vasc Biol 2000; 20(3):836–45.

79. Nakazawa G, Otsuka F, Nakano M, et al. The pathology of neoatherosclerosis in human coronary implants bare-metal and drug-eluting stents. J Am Coll Cardiol 2011;57(11):1314–22.

80. Joner M, Nakazawa G, Finn AV, et al. Endothelial cell recovery between comparator polymer-based drug-eluting stents. J Am Coll Cardiol 2008;52(5): 333–42.

81. Nakazawa G, Vorpahl M, Finn AV, et al. One step forward and two steps back with drug-eluting-stents: from preventing restenosis to causing late thrombosis and nouveau atherosclerosis. JACC Cardiovasc Imaging 2009;2(5):625–8.

82. Shankman LS, Gomez D, Cherepanova OA, et al. KLF4-dependent phenotypic modulation of smooth muscle cells has a key role in atherosclerotic plaque pathogenesis. Nat Med 2015;21(6): 628–37.

83. Buja LM. Vascular responses to percutaneous coronary intervention with bare-metal stents and drug-eluting stents: a perspective based on insights from pathological and clinical studies. J Am Coll Cardiol 2011;57(11):1323–6.

84. Stone GW, Ellis SG, Colombo A, et al. Offsetting impact of thrombosis and restenosis on the occurrence of death and myocardial infarction after paclitaxel-eluting and bare metal stent implantation. Circulation 2007;115(22):2842–7.

85. Wenaweser P, Daemen J, Zwahlen M, et al. Incidence and correlates of drug-eluting stent thrombosis in routine clinical practice. 4-year results from a large 2-institutional cohort study. J Am Coll Cardiol 2008;52(14):1134–40.

86. Natsuaki M, Morimoto T, Furukawa Y, et al. Late adverse events after implantation of sirolimus-eluting stent and bare-metal stent: long-term (5-7 years) follow-up of the Coronary Revascularization Demonstrating Outcome study-Kyoto registry Cohort-2. Circ Cardiovasc Interv 2014;7(2):168–79.

87. Yamaji K, Kimura T, Morimoto T, et al. Very long-term (15 to 20 years) clinical and angiographic outcome after coronary bare metal stent implantation. Circ Cardiovasc Interv 2010;3(5):468–75.

88. Joner M, Finn AV, Farb A, et al. Pathology of drug-eluting stents in humans: delayed healing and late thrombotic risk. J Am Coll Cardiol 2006; 48(1):193–202.

89. Nakazawa G, Finn AV, Vorpahl M, et al. Incidence and predictors of drug-eluting stent fracture in human coronary artery a pathologic analysis. J Am Coll Cardiol 2009;54(21):1924–31.

90. Taniwaki M, Windecker S, Raber L. Neoatherosclerosis as reason for stent failures beyond 5 years after drug-eluting stent implantation. Eur Heart J 2014;35(29):1980.

91. Takano M, Yamamoto M, Inami S, et al. Appearance of lipid-laden intima and neovascularization after implantation of bare-metal stents extended late-phase observation by intracoronary optical coherence tomography. J Am Coll Cardiol 2009; 55(1):26–32.

92. Holmes DR Jr, Kereiakes DJ, Garg S, et al. Stent thrombosis. J Am Coll Cardiol 2010;56(17):1357–65.

93. Finn AV, Joner M, Nakazawa G, et al. Pathological correlates of late drug-eluting stent thrombosis: strut coverage as a marker of endothelialization. Circulation 2007;115(18):2435–41.

94. Raber L, Magro M, Stefanini GG, et al. Very late coronary stent thrombosis of a newer-generation everolimus-eluting stent compared with early-generation drug-eluting stents: a prospective cohort study. Circulation 2012;125(9):1110–21.

95. Daemen J, Wenaweser P, Tsuchida K, et al. Early and late coronary stent thrombosis of sirolimus-eluting and paclitaxel-eluting stents in routine clinical practice: data from a large two-institutional cohort study. Lancet 2007;369(9562):667–78.

96. Babapulle MN, Joseph L, Belisle P, et al. A hierarchical Bayesian meta-analysis of randomised clinical trials of drug-eluting stents. Lancet 2004;364(9434):583–91.

97. Moreno R, Fernandez C, Hernandez R, et al. Drug-eluting stent thrombosis: results from a pooled analysis including 10 randomized studies. J Am Coll Cardiol 2005;45(6):954–9.

98. Bavry AA, Kumbhani DJ, Helton TJ, et al. What is the risk of stent thrombosis associated with the use of paclitaxel-eluting stents for percutaneous coronary intervention?: a meta-analysis. J Am Coll Cardiol 2005;45(6):941–6.

99. Stone GW, Moses JW, Ellis SG, et al. Safety and efficacy of sirolimus- and paclitaxel-eluting coronary stents. N Engl J Med 2007;356(10):998–1008.

100. Awata M, Kotani J, Uematsu M, et al. Serial angioscopic evidence of incomplete neointimal coverage after sirolimus-eluting stent implantation: comparison with bare-metal stents. Circulation 2007;116(8):910–6.

101. Wakabayashi K, Mintz GS, Weissman NJ, et al. Impact of drug-eluting stents on distal vessels. Circ Cardiovasc Interv 2012;5(2):211–9.

102. Wakabayashi K, Waksman R, Weissman NJ. Edge effect from drug-eluting stents as assessed with serial intravascular ultrasound: a systematic review. Circ Cardiovasc Interv 2012;5(2):305–11.

103. Kedhi E, Joesoef KS, McFadden E, et al. Second-generation everolimus-eluting and paclitaxel-eluting stents in real-life practice (COMPARE): a randomised trial. Lancet 2010;375(9710):201–9.

104. Smits PC, Kedhi E, Royaards KJ, et al. 2-year follow-up of a randomized controlled trial of everolimus- and paclitaxel-eluting stents for coronary revascularization in daily practice. COMPARE (Comparison of the everolimus eluting XIENCE-V stent with the paclitaxel eluting TAXUS LIBERTE stent in all-comers: a randomized open label trial). J Am Coll Cardiol 2011;58(1):11–8.

105. Stone GW, Rizvi A, Sudhir K, et al. Randomized comparison of everolimus- and paclitaxel-eluting stents. 2-year follow-up from the SPIRIT (Clinical Evaluation of the XIENCE V Everolimus Eluting Coronary Stent System) IV trial. J Am Coll Cardiol 2011;58(1):19–25.

106. Palmerini T, Biondi-Zoccai G, Della Riva D, et al. Stent thrombosis with drug-eluting and bare-metal stents: evidence from a comprehensive network meta-analysis. Lancet 2012;379(9824):1393–402.

107. Bangalore S, Kumar S, Fusaro M, et al. Short- and long-term outcomes with drug-eluting and bare-metal coronary stents: a mixed-treatment comparison analysis of 117 762 patient-years of follow-up from randomized trials. Circulation 2012;125(23):2873–91.

108. Tada T, Byrne RA, Simunovic I, et al. Risk of stent thrombosis among bare-metal stents, first-generation drug-eluting stents, and second-generation drug-eluting stents: results from a registry of 18,334 patients. JACC Cardiovasc Interv 2013;6(12):1267–74.

109. Cassese S, Byrne RA, Tada T, et al. Incidence and predictors of restenosis after coronary stenting in 10 004 patients with surveillance angiography. Heart 2014;100(2):153–9.

110. Lee SY, Hur SH, Lee SG, et al. Optical coherence tomographic observation of in-stent neoatherosclerosis in lesions with more than 50% neointimal area stenosis after second-generation drug-eluting stent implantation. Circ Cardiovasc Interv 2015;8(2):e001878.

111. Brener SJ, Kereiakes DJ, Simonton CA, et al. Everolimus-eluting stents in patients undergoing percutaneous coronary intervention: final 3-year results of the Clinical Evaluation of the XIENCE V Everolimus Eluting Coronary Stent System in the Treatment of Subjects With de Novo Native Coronary Artery Lesions trial. Am Heart J 2013;166(6):1035–42.

112. Lee JM, Park KW, Han JK, et al. Three-year patient-related and stent-related outcomes of second-generation everolimus-eluting Xience V stents versus zotarolimus-eluting resolute stents in real-world practice (from the Multicenter Prospective EXCELLENT and RESOLUTE-Korea Registries). Am J Cardiol 2014;114(9):1329–38.

113. Camenzind E, Wijns W, Mauri L, et al. Stent thrombosis and major clinical events at 3 years after zotarolimus-eluting or sirolimus-eluting coronary stent implantation: a randomised, multicentre, open-label, controlled trial. Lancet 2012;380(9851):1396–405.

114. Inoue T, Shite J, Yoon J, et al. Optical coherence evaluation of everolimus-eluting stents 8 months after implantation. Heart 2011;97(17):1379–84.

115. Otsuka F, Vorpahl M, Nakano M, et al. Pathology of second-generation everolimus-eluting stents versus first-generation sirolimus- and paclitaxel-eluting stents in humans. Circulation 2014;129(2):211–23.

116. Yonetsu T, Kim JS, Kato K, et al. Comparison of incidence and time course of neoatherosclerosis between bare metal stents and drug-eluting stents using optical coherence tomography. Am J Cardiol 2012;110(7):933–9.

117. Taniwaki M, Windecker S, Zaugg S, et al. The association between in-stent neoatherosclerosis and native coronary artery disease progression: a long-term angiographic and optical coherence tomography cohort study. Eur Heart J 2015;36(32):2167–76.

118. Iijima R, Araki T, Nagashima Y, et al. Incidence and predictors of the late catch-up phenomenon after drug-eluting stent implantation. Int J Cardiol 2013;168(3):2588–92.

119. Nakazawa G, Yazdani SK, Finn AV, et al. Pathological findings at bifurcation lesions: the impact of flow distribution on atherosclerosis and arterial healing after stent implantation. J Am Coll Cardiol 2010;55(16):1679–87.

120. Wilson GJ, Nakazawa G, Schwartz RS, et al. Comparison of inflammatory response after implantation of sirolimus- and paclitaxel-eluting stents in porcine coronary arteries. Circulation 2009;120(2):141–9, 1-2.

121. Finn AV, Kolodgie FD, Harnek J, et al. Differential response of delayed healing and persistent inflammation at sites of overlapping sirolimus- or paclitaxel-eluting stents. Circulation 2005;112(2):270–8.

122. Finn AV, Nakazawa G, Joner M, et al. Vascular responses to drug eluting stents: importance of delayed healing. Arterioscler Thromb Vasc Biol 2007;27(7):1500–10.

123. Byrne RA. Bioresorbable vascular scaffolds–will promise become reality? N Engl J Med 2015;373(20):1969–71.

124. Verheye S, Ormiston JA, Stewart J, et al. A next-generation bioresorbable coronary scaffold system: from bench to first clinical evaluation: 6- and 12-month clinical and multimodality imaging results. JACC Cardiovasc Interv 2014;7(1):89–99.

125. Serruys PW, Ormiston JA, Onuma Y, et al. A bioabsorbable everolimus-eluting coronary stent system (ABSORB): 2-year outcomes and results from multiple imaging methods. Lancet 2009;373(9667):897–910.

126. Ellis SG, Kereiakes DJ, Metzger DC, et al. Everolimus-eluting bioresorbable scaffolds for coronary artery disease. N Engl J Med 2015;373(20):1905–15.

127. Miyazaki T, Panoulas VF, Sato K, et al. Acute stent thrombosis of a bioresorbable vascular scaffold implanted for ST-segment elevation myocardial infarction. Int J Cardiol 2014;174(2):e72–4.

128. Karanasos A, van Geuns RJ, Zijlstra F, et al. Very late bioresorbable scaffold thrombosis after discontinuation of dual antiplatelet therapy. Eur Heart J 2014;35(27):1781.

129. Sanchez OD, Yahagi K, Byrne RA, et al. Pathological aspects of bioresorbable stent implantation. EuroIntervention 2015;11(Suppl V):V159–65.

130. Otsuka F, Pacheco E, Perkins LE, et al. Long-term safety of an everolimus-eluting bioresorbable vascular scaffold and the cobalt-chromium XIENCE V stent in a porcine coronary artery model. Circ Cardiovasc Interv 2014;7(3):330–42.

131. Danson E, Bhindi R, Hansen P. Follow-up evaluation of unapposed bioresorbable vascular scaffold at a coronary bifurcation using optical coherence tomography. Int J Cardiol 2014;177(2):e84–6.

132. Simsek C, Karanasos A, Magro M, et al. Long-term invasive follow-up of the everolimus-eluting bioresorbable vascular scaffold: five-year results of multiple invasive imaging modalities. EuroIntervention 2016;11(9):996–1003.

Coronary Stent Failure
Fracture, Compression, Recoil, and Prolapse

Dominik M. Wiktor, MD, Stephen W. Waldo, MD,
Ehrin J. Armstrong, MD, MSc*

KEYWORDS

- Stent fracture • Longitudinal stent deformation • Stent recoil • Plaque prolapse

---

KEY POINTS

- Despite significant improvements in coronary stent designs, several important mechanisms of coronary stent failure must be recognized.
- Stent fracture is more common in the right coronary artery, in tortuous lesions, and with stiffer stent scaffold designs.
- Longitudinal stent deformation occurs owing to compression or elongation of a stent and is more likely to occur in stents with 2 or fewer connectors.
- Stent recoil results in suboptimal stent cross-sectional area, and may be more common with bioresorbable scaffolds.

INTRODUCTION

Since the development of balloon-expandable coronary stents, numerous engineering innovations have improved the intraprocedural and long-term outcomes of percutaneous coronary intervention. Despite these innovations, there remain several, albeit uncommon, mechanisms of stent failure that are associated with adverse clinical outcomes. In this paper, we review the major mechanisms of coronary stent failure, including stent fracture, longitudinal deformation, recoil, and plaque prolapse. We also discuss failure mechanisms that are specific to and more common with bioresorbable vascular scaffolds (BVS).

CORONARY STENT FRACTURE

Although less common with current generation of drug-eluting stents, stent fracture was a frequent complication of early generation

sirolimus-eluting stents.[1–8] Despite improvements in stent design, stent fracture can still occur with the current of generation drug-eluting stents, with an observed incidence between 0.8% and 8.0%.[9] This large range of incidence is likely multifactorial, owing to the majority of data being derived from single center observational studies, the variability in definition of stent fracture, and the variability of the screening tool used. For example, intravascular ultrasound (IVUS) examination and optical coherence tomography have a much greater sensitivity in detecting stent factures compared with conventional angiography.[10,11] Autopsy studies have suggested that the rate of coronary stent fracture approaches 29%, but only the most severe fractures are associated with evident intracoronary pathologic changes.[12]

Mechanisms of Coronary Stent Fracture

Several factors are associated with an increased incidence of coronary stent fracture. These

---

Disclosures/Conflicts of Interest: E.J. Armstrong is a consultant/advisory board member to Abbott Vascular, Medtronic, Merck, and Spectranetics. All other authors report no conflicts of interest.
Division of Cardiology, VA Eastern Colorado Healthcare System, University of Colorado, Denver, CO, USA
* Corresponding author. Denver VA Medical Center, 1055 Clermont Street, Denver, CO 80220.
E-mail address: ehrin.armstrong@gmail.com

Intervent Cardiol Clin 5 (2016) 405–414
http://dx.doi.org/10.1016/j.iccl.2016.03.004
2211-7458/16/$ – see front matter Published by Elsevier Inc.

factors include the target vessel, the type of stent, use of overlapping stents, and vessel angulation. Larger stent size may be associated with a lower risk of stent fracture.[13] Importantly, there is no relationship between stent deployment inflation pressures or the routine use of postdilation and the risk of subsequent stent fracture.

The right coronary artery (RCA) is the most common coronary vessel associated with development of stent fracture, with up to 50% of reported stent fractures occurring in the RCA. The anatomic location, angulation, and significant motion of the RCA during the cardiac cycle all play a role in the generation of torsion forces, which may predispose patients to stent fracture. In addition to the RCA, stents placed in saphenous vein grafts are also associated with a higher rate of fracture than those in the left coronary circulation.[14] The mechanisms specific to stent fracture in saphenous vein grafts are unclear, but may also be related to graft movement with the cardiac cycle, especially for stents that are placed at the ostium of a vein graft. Interestingly, the majority of bare metal stent fractures have been reported in saphenous vein grafts, with few published data on bare metal stent fracture in native coronary arteries.[15–17]

Coronary vessel tortuosity and angulation also play an important role in stent fracture. Observational studies have implicated both vessel tortuosity and extreme angulation in the development of a fracture.[7,14,18] These studies suggest that the majority of stent fractures occur when stent angulation exceeds 45°, with 1 study describing greater than 90% of stent fractures occurring in vessels where stent angulation exceeds 75°.[13]

The risk of stent fracture was clearly greater in early generation self-expanding stents as compared with contemporary platforms. However, there are limited clinical and laboratory data regarding the relative incidence, which suggests that even newer generation drug-eluting stents are prone to fracture.[3,19] In 1 series investigating fracture of platinum-chromium everolimus-eluting stents, the reported rate of stent fracture was 1.7%.[3]

In addition to clinical studies, laboratory bench tests evaluating the impact of repetitive bending motion on stent fracture have been performed and corroborate some conclusions garnered from clinical studies. Namely, in vitro studies have shown that vessel motion and angulation play an important role in stent fracture. Additionally, increased stent rigidity (determined primarily by the number of strut connectors) is related to an increased likelihood of stent fracture.[19]

Classification of Coronary Stent Fractures

Because a stent fracture can be detected by various imaging modalities, a single unified classification system for stent fracture does not exist. The most frequently used classification stratifies fracture type by the number and extent of fractured struts (Table 1).[12] In this angiography-based definition, stent fractures are graded as types I through V. Type I fractures are associated with the presence of a single fractured strut; type II fractures involved 2 or more struts, but without stent deformation; type III fractures involve associated stent deformation; type IV fractures comprise transection of the stent without a gap; and type V fractures involve transection with an associated gap in the stent.

In comparison with an angiography-based definition, classification of stent fracture by IVUS is predicated on the presence or absence of aneurysm formation. This is a binary system, with a type I stent fracture not associated with aneurysm and a type II stent fracture associated with aneurysm.[10] In this schema, it is thought that type I fractures are acute and related to bending forces in coronary vessels. In contrast, type II fractures may be related to the biological effects of eluted drugs, with positive vessel remodeling leading to late stent malapposition, aneurysm formation, and stent fracture.[20] Additionally, systems exist for classification of fracture type by computed tomography, although these systems are less often of clinical usefulness in the catheterization laboratory.

Clinical Implications of Coronary Stent Fracture

The presence of stent fracture has clearly been implicated in both in-stent restenosis (ISR) and stent thrombosis with resultant acute coronary syndrome (ACS). The likelihood of superimposed ISR on stent fracture ranges from 15% to nearly 90% in the available literature, with rates of target lesion revascularization of nearly

Table 1 Angiographic classification of coronary stent fractures	
Type I	Single Strut Fracture
Type II	≥2 Strut Fracture
Type III	≥2 Strut Fracture with deformation
Type IV	Fracture with transection but no gap
Type V	Fracture with a gap

50% as compared with 11% in non–fracture-related ISR.[1,5,13,18]

The mechanisms for clinically relevant ISR associated with stent fracture are incompletely understood. However, 1 theory is that stent fracture leads to incomplete or inefficient local drug delivery in the areas where the stent is disrupted.[14] This abnormality may lead to local neointimal hyperplasia and luminal area loss. The presence of displaced struts may also result in repetitive vessel trauma, with a subsequent activation of the coagulation cascade and increased platelet activation.

In addition to the subacute issues related to ISR, there have been several reported cases of stent thrombosis and ACS associated with stent fracture. Although the reported risk of cardiac death in patients with ACS related to stent fracture is low, caution must be urged because stent fracture in patients with ACS and prior percutaneous coronary intervention is likely underrecognized.[21,22]

Treatment of Coronary Stent Fracture

Although there is little evidence to guide clinical care for patients with stent fracture, several management strategies have been proposed. In patients with mild stent fracture and no ISR, it may be reasonable to continue a longer duration dual antiplatelet therapy given the associated risk of restenosis and stent thrombosis.[23] In patients with more severe stent fracture and flow-limiting ISR, the use of additional overlapping stents has been used with reasonable success (**Figs. 1** and **2**). In patients with more significant stent fracture and no evidence of ISR, the optimal management has not been clearly defined.

Summary

Intracoronary stent fracture is a relatively uncommon, although likely an underrecognized, mechanism for both clinically relevant ISR and ACS. Early generation sirolimus-eluting stents were associated with a higher rate of stent fracture, likely related to increased "stiffness" of the strut connectors in this platform, although fractures have also been observed in contemporary stent designs. The optimal treatment for stent fracture has not been elucidated and several approaches have been proposed with relatively limited data on outcomes of these strategies.

LONGITUDINAL STENT DEFORMATION

The development and clinical use of coronary stents with thinner struts, fewer strut connectors, and more flexible alloys (eg, cobalt chromium, platinum chromium) has led to greater deliverability of these platforms compared with early generation stainless steel stents. These advances, however, may also be associated with a decrease in longitudinal strength. Several case reports, observational studies, and bench tests have highlighted the incidence, mechanisms and clinical impact of longitudinal stent deformation (LSD), defined as either shortening or elongation along the longitudinal axis of these more deliverable platforms.

The vast majority of data on LSD come after 2010, when more deliverable and thinner strutted platforms with fewer connectors were

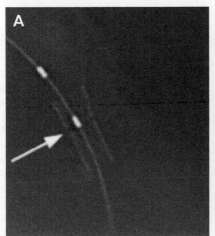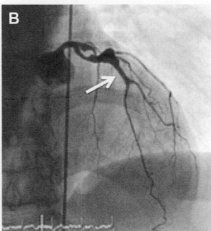

Fig. 1. Stent fracture. A type V fracture (complete stent disarticulation with a gap) is apparent in the proximal segment of the stent (*A, arrow*) with no angiographic evidence of flow limitation or in-stent restenosis (ISR) (*B, arrow*). Given the lack of ISR or other clinical sequelae, this stent fracture was managed conservatively.

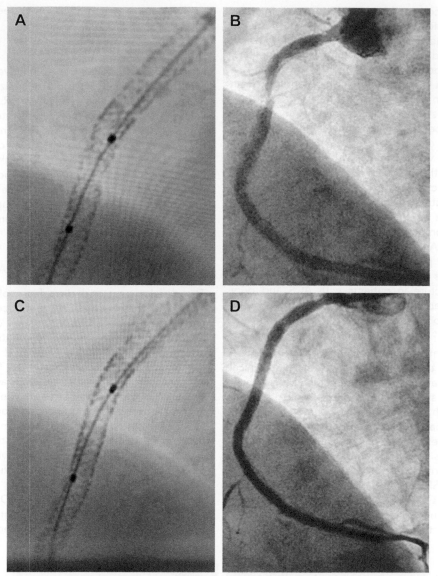

Fig. 2. Stent fracture with associated in-stent restenosis. A type V stent fracture (*A*) with resultant severe in-stent restenosis (*B*). Given the restenosis, this lesion was treated with placement of an overlapping layer of stent (*C*) with excellent angiographic result (*D*).

introduced, most specifically the Promus Element platform, which has been the most widely studied and reported platform in which LSD is observed both in clinical practice and on the bench.[24–33]

Mechanisms and Classification of Longitudinal Stent Deformation

There are 2 major mechanisms leading to balloon expandable coronary stent LSD: (1) intrinsic stent deformation related to balloon expansion and (2) extrinsic influences such vessel characteristics or trauma related to interventional equipment. Several studies have found that all balloon expandable coronary stents are deformable to some degree along the longitudinal axis. Invariably in bench testing, if force is applied to the longitudinal axis of a balloon expandable coronary stent, there will be deformation to varying degrees. Another fairly consistent finding among these tests relates to the increased deformability of stents constructed with only 2 intercrown connectors (ie, Element, Driver), although there is little difference among other platforms that use more than 2 connectors.[25,30,31,34]

Most commonly, the bench tests used to assess LSD apply longitudinal force in a circumferential manner to stent platforms to assess for deformation. This method is quantitative, but incompletely reflects clinical practice. Ormiston and colleagues[30] have reported a second-generation bench test that applies asymmetric force to stent platforms, thus more closely replicating the stent trauma that can occur in clinical practice. The results of this technique have demonstrated that the mechanism of failure in LSD is multifaceted. Although essentially all cases involve stent compression along the longitudinal axis, stent strut separation (pseudofracture), and intrusion into the lumen is also observed, highlighting the complex geometric alterations that may distort the overall 3-dimensional stent architecture.[30]

In addition to issues related to stent design and construction, there are several anatomic and lesion-specific considerations that increase the likelihood of LSD. More complex coronary artery disease, including the presence of lesion calcification, longer lesion length, and vessel tortuosity can each predispose to LSD. Additionally, LSD is observed more frequently when treating bifurcation or aortoostial (specifically left main coronary artery) coronary artery disease.[26,35] In the case of bifurcation disease, the increased risk of LSD is likely related to the multiple device manipulations that are necessary to treat bifurcation lesions, as well as the increased stent angulation when deployed across a bifurcation. In the case of aortoostial lesions, guide catheter interaction with the proximal edge can predispose to compression and LSD. Severe vessel calcification and tortuosity along with long lesion length have been observed commonly in cases of LSD.[26,35]

There are 3 patterns of LSD as defined in an IVUS study by Inaba and colleagues[35] as follows: (1) deformation with intrastent wrinkling and overlapping of the proximal and distal stent fragments within a single stent (most common), (2) deformation with elongation, and (3) deformation with shortening. Expanding further on available data, Mamas and Williams published a proposed classification system (Table 2), which categorizes LSD based on location within the stent along with the proposed mechanism of deformation. In general, proximal deformation most frequently occurs owing to interaction with a guide or guide catheter extension, whereas distal deformation is likely related to stent compression while withdrawing a secondary device.

Although the clinically apparent incidence of coronary stent LSD is low (<1%), studies that have investigated LSD using advanced imaging modalities have reported higher rates, highlighting the potential issues of using only

Table 2
Classification and proposed mechanisms of longitudinal stent deformation

Stent Location	Proposed Mechanisms
Proximal	Guide catheter compression Guide extension compression Passing a secondary device into stent (eg, balloon, filter retrieval)
Distal	Withdrawal of secondary device through stent (eg, balloon, intravascular ultrasound catheter)
Any location	Withdrawal of deflated postdilation balloons

angiography as a means for detecting LSD. In one study by Inaba and associates,[35] only 3 of 17 IVUS-confirmed LSD cases (17.6%) were observed by angiography.

Clinical Impact and Treatment of Longitudinal Stent Deformation

Despite the increased awareness of LSD since the introduction of less rigid stent platforms, the incidence of clinically relevant LSD as a complication of percutaneous coronary intervention remains rare. There have been only a handful of adverse clinical outcomes related to LSD reported in the literature to date, with studies from the MAUDE database providing the greatest insight into the clinical impact of this problem.[26,27,33,36] These complications have been related to acute stent thrombosis, guidewire/balloon entrapment and vascular complications. The presence of LSD increases the risk of stent thrombosis and ISR based on these reports; however, the incidence remains low.

Although no formal outcomes studies have been published, observational data have suggested that treating LSD with postdilation and implantation of overlapping stents to cover the area of LSD is reasonable.[26,29,34–36] There have also been reports of patients requiring emergent coronary artery bypass grafting to remove entrapped equipment from deformed stents.[26] Additionally, there has been limited experience with rotational atherectomy to "ablate" the deformed stent and facilitate placement of additional stents (Fig. 3). These reports highlight the lack of data regarding optimal treatment of LSD.

Summary

All balloon expandable intracoronary stents are prone to longitudinal deformation with applied force; however, stents with 2 or more connectors

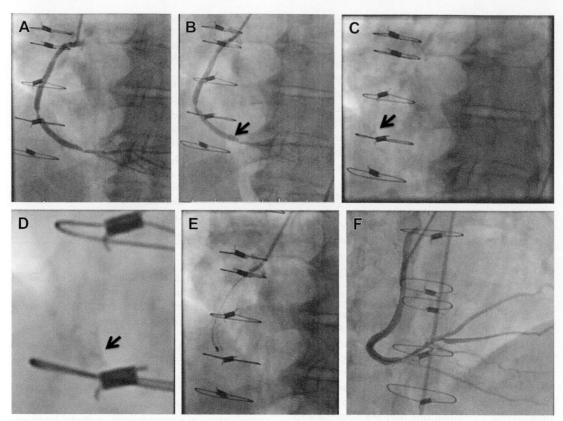

Fig. 3. Longitudinal stent deformation. (A) A severe stenosis was noted in the mid segment of a saphenous vein graft to the distal right coronary artery. (B) A distal embolic protection filter (arrow) was placed during percutaneous coronary intervention. (C) After stent placement, the filter was removed but caught on the distal edge of the stent, causing longitudinal stent deformation and the presence of a "double density" on the angiogram (arrow). (D) Magnified view of the longitudinal deformation (arrow). (E) Owing to difficulty with delivering devices through the site of deformation, rotational atherectomy was performed to obliterate the site of stent deformation. (F) Final angiographic result after subsequent angioplasty and repeat stent implantation.

seem to be the least resistant to longitudinal forces. LSD is an uncommon mechanism of failure of balloon expandable intracoronary stent failure. Despite this, certain lesion subsets place stents at high likelihood of LSD, namely aortoostial disease, heavily calcified and tortuous lesions, and longer lesions. The optimal treatment for clinically significant LSD has not been studied; however, the use of postdilation balloons and additional stents has been reported.

STENT RECOIL

Stent recoil, defined as a loss in cross-sectional area (CSA) and failure to achieve nominal CSA after full expansion of a stent, was recognized early after the advent of intracoronary balloon expandable stents.[37–40] Early metallic stents were prone to acute recoil after balloon expansion, resulting in CSA loss of anywhere between 15% and 50%. Recoil was especially prominent in the coil-type stent designs when compared with

the early slotted tube–type stents. The issue was primarily dealt with by employing aggressive postdilation to achieve nominal CSA after recoil.[37,38] Stent recoil is currently less of a concern with the current generation of cobalt chromium and platinum chromium stents, but remains an area of concern with the introduction of BVS to clinical practice.[41]

With the introduction of thinner strutted platforms, there were concerns regarding a possible reduction in radial strength. Based on retrospective clinical studies using IVUS to measure postdelivery CSA, there does not seem to be a loss in radial strength or risk of acute recoil with current generation thinner struts.[42,43] With the introduction of BVS, there has been a focus of both acute and chronic stent recoil given the properties of these platforms.[41,44]

Acute Versus Chronic Stent Recoil
Acute stent recoil, defined as CSA loss immediately after adequate balloon expansion, has

been described as a mechanism for early stent malapposition in relation to other issues, such as vessel remodeling after percutaneous coronary intervention.[45] This issue seems to be less of a problem with current generation stent platforms, with acute CSA loss in the single digit percent ranges and up to 10% in cobalt–chromium platforms.[46]

Chronic recoil may be related to late lumen area loss and ISR in the current generation of metallic stents; however, the percent CSA loss is reported to be only on the order of 4% in contemporary metallic stents. Studies have reported a higher magnitude of late CSA loss in BVS (approximately 7%) as compared with metallic stents. There may also be a decrease in radial strength over time as bioresorption of the stent scaffold takes place, which may be in part related to the late loss in CSA. However, this does not seem to translate into meaningful differences in clinical outcomes in BVS versus metallic stents.[41,44]

Clinical Impact and Treatment of Stent Recoil

The clinical impact of acute or chronic stent recoil is related to failure to achieve appropriate CSA, with an attendant increased risk of subsequent restenosis or stent thrombosis. Certain lesion characteristics predispose to recoil, with stents placed in fibronecrotic plaque being more prone to recoil than those deployed in calcified plaque.[41] Although clinically meaningful recoil has been reported, its incidence is exceedingly low. Several means of rectifying the CSA loss in these situations have been reported, including aggressive postdilation and placement of a second stent within the lumen of the initial stent that developed recoil without any significant untoward events reported.[44,45,47]

TISSUE PROLAPSE

Tissue prolapse (TP), defined as intrusion of plaque or tissue between stent struts into the vessel lumen, has long been recognized after coronary stent implantation.[48–51] Some data have suggested that tissue prolapse may increase the risk of stent thrombosis and markers of myocardial injury; however, no clear association with poor long-term outcomes has been observed.[49,52,53] Recent reports corroborate prior findings of a higher incidence of TP when optical coherence tomography is used as the screening tool and highlights the debate regarding the clinical significance of this finding.[54] Targeted treatment of TP has been attempted, but without any definite impact on clinically relevant endpoints.[55,56]

Incidence and Causes of Tissue Prolapse

The incidence of TP depends highly on the imaging modality used. The observed incidence of TP in IVUS studies ranges from 25% to nearly 60%.[48–50,52,53,57,58] However, when optical coherence tomography is used, the incidence of TP has been reported to be greater than 95%.[51,54]

Stent type influences the degree of tissue or plaque prolapse, with early generation stainless steel stents demonstrating less tissue prolapse as compared with newer generation metal alloy stents.[49,50,57] There is also a higher observed rate of TP in noncalcified lesions, longer lesions, small lumen diameter, angulated lesions, and in infarct-related arteries.[48,49,57]

Clinical Impact and Treatment of Tissue Prolapse

The impact of TP has been measured both biochemically and in the context of major adverse cardiovascular events (MACE). Although studies have demonstrated an absolute increase in creatine kinase levels in patients in whom TP is observed, there seems to be no correlation with late outcomes including MACE.[49,53] Other studies have suggested a possible increased risk of stent thrombosis in the presence of TP, although overall adverse events are not significantly greater.[52]

Given the increased incidence of myonecrosis in patients with TP, and increased risk for TP and distal embolization in patients with ST-segment elevation myocardial infarction, a novel micronet mesh–covered stent, MGuard (InspireMD, Tel Aviv, Israel), was developed to trap atheroma and thrombus and thereby prevent embolization. In a clinical trial evaluating the efficacy of the MGuard stent, the device had higher rates of complete ST-segment resolution and improved epicardial flow as assessed by Thrombolysis In Myocardial Infarction classification as compared with controls. Despite these encouraging early outcomes, there was no difference in mortality and MACE at 30 days.[55] However, there was a higher risk of MACE with MGuard at 1 year, primarily driven by target lesion revascularization, with no difference in rates of myocardial infarction or death.[56]

Summary

TP is a common problem observed after implantation of balloon expandable coronary stents. Despite the high incidence of TP, the clinical impact of this problem is limited, however it is important to recognize that stent thrombosis rates and the degree of myonecrosis may be increased in patients with TP without definite long-term implications on MACE.

SUMMARY

Contemporary stent failure is a relatively rare occurrence that is frequently insignificant clinically. Stent fracture and recoil are relatively uncommon with the current generation of stents, although they may become an issue with the wider adoption of bioasborbable scaffolds. Longitudinal deformation and tissue prolapse can occur, especially with more flexible and open cell stent designs, although optimal management is less clear. As newer generation bioresorbable scaffolds and other novel approaches to percutaneous coronary intervention are developed, it will be important to continue to analyze mechanisms of stent failure. Additionally, dedicated studies with newer imaging modalities such as optical coherence tomography may provide novel insights into the mechanical mechanisms of stent failure.

REFERENCES

1. Aoki J, Nakazawa G, Tanabe K, et al. Incidence and clinical impact of coronary stent fracture after sirolimus-eluting stent implantation. Catheter Cardiovasc Interv 2007;69(3):380–6.

2. Ohya M, Kadota K, Tada T, et al. Stent fracture after sirolimus-eluting stent implantation: 8-year clinical outcomes. Circ Cardiovasc Interv 2015;8(8): e002664.

3. Kuramitsu S, Hiromasa T, Enomoto S, et al. Incidence and clinical impact of stent fracture after PROMUS element platinum chromium everolimus-eluting stent implantation. JACC Cardiovasc Interv 2015;8(9):1180–8.

4. Chinikar M, Sadeghipour P. Coronary stent fracture: a recently appreciated phenomenon with clinical relevance. Curr Cardiol Rev 2014;10(4):349–54.

5. Umeda H, Kawai T, Misumida N, et al. Impact of sirolimus-eluting stent fracture on 4-year clinical outcomes. Circ Cardiovasc Interv 2011;4(4):349–54.

6. Canan T, Lee MS. Drug-eluting stent fracture: incidence, contributing factors, and clinical implications. Catheter Cardiovasc Interv 2010;75(2):237–45.

7. Chakravarty T, White AJ, Buch M, et al. Meta-analysis of incidence, clinical characteristics and implications of stent fracture. Am J Cardiol 2010; 106(8):1075–80.

8. Carter AJ. Drug-eluting stent fracture promise and performance. J Am Coll Cardiol 2009;54(21):1932–4.

9. Williams PD. Stent fracture with contemporary coronary stent platforms. EuroIntervention 2014;10(5): 651–2.

10. Doi H, Maehara A, Mintz GS, et al. Intravascular ultrasound findings of stent fractures in patients with Sirolimus- and Paclitaxel-eluting stents. Am J Cardiol 2010;106(7):952–7.

11. Yamada KP, Koizumi T, Yamaguchi H, et al. Serial angiographic and intravascular ultrasound analysis of late stent strut fracture of sirolimus-eluting stents in native coronary arteries. Int J Cardiol 2008;130(2): 255–9.

12. Nakazawa G, Finn AV, Vorpahl M, et al. Incidence and predictors of drug-eluting stent fracture in human coronary artery a pathologic analysis. J Am Coll Cardiol 2009;54(21):1924–31.

13. Shaikh F, Maddikunta R, Djelmami-Hani M, et al. Stent fracture, an incidental finding or a significant marker of clinical in-stent restenosis? Catheter Cardiovasc Interv 2008;71(5):614–8.

14. Lee MS, Jurewitz D, Aragon J, et al. Stent fracture associated with drug-eluting stents: clinical characteristics and implications. Catheter Cardiovasc Interv 2007;69(3):387–94.

15. Dorsch MF, Seidelin PH, Blackman DJ. Stent fracture and collapse in a saphenous vein graft causing occlusive restenosis. J Invasive Cardiol 2006;18(4): E137–9.

16. Chowdhury PS, Ramos RG. Images in clinical medicine. Coronary-stent fracture. N Engl J Med 2002; 347(8):581.

17. Koh TW, Mathur A. Coronary stent fracture in a saphenous vein graft to right coronary artery–successful treatment by the novel use of the Jomed coronary stent graft: case report and review of the literature. Int J Cardiol 2007;119(2):e43–5.

18. Umeda H, Gochi T, Iwase M, et al. Frequency, predictors and outcome of stent fracture after sirolimus-eluting stent implantation. Int J Cardiol 2009;133(3):321–6.

19. Ormiston JA, Webber B, Ubod B, et al. Coronary stent durability and fracture: an independent bench comparison of six contemporary designs using a repetitive bend test. EuroIntervention 2015;10(12): 1449–55.

20. Doi H, Maehara A, Mintz GS, et al. Classification and potential mechanisms of intravascular ultrasound patterns of stent fracture. Am J Cardiol 2009;103(6):818–23.

21. Amico F, Geraci S, Tamburino C. Acute coronary syndrome due to early multiple and complete fractures in sirolimus-eluting stent: a case report and brief literature review. Catheter Cardiovasc Interv 2013;81(1):52–6.

22. Chhatriwalla AK, Cam A, Unzek S, et al. Drug-eluting stent fracture and acute coronary syndrome. Cardiovasc Revasc Med 2009;10(3): 166–71.

23. Lee SE, Jeong MH, Kim IS, et al. Clinical outcomes and optimal treatment for stent fracture after

drug-eluting stent implantation. J Cardiol 2009; 53(3):422–8.

24. Leibundgut G, Gick M, Toma A, et al. Longitudinal compression of the platinum-chromium everolimus-eluting stent during coronary implantation: predisposing mechanical properties, incidence, and predictors in a large patient cohort. Catheter Cardiovasc Interv 2013;81(5):E206–14.

25. Prabhu S, Schikorr T, Mahmoud T, et al. Engineering assessment of the longitudinal compression behaviour of contemporary coronary stents. EuroIntervention 2012;8(2):275–81.

26. Mamas MA, Foin N, Abunassar C, et al. Stent fracture: insights on mechanisms, treatments, and outcomes from the food and drug administration manufacturer and user facility device experience database. Catheter Cardiovasc Interv 2014;83(7): E251–9.

27. Williams PD, Mamas MA, Morgan KP, et al. Longitudinal stent deformation: a retrospective analysis of frequency and mechanisms. EuroIntervention 2012;8(2):267–74.

28. Hanratty CG, Walsh SJ. Longitudinal compression: a "new" complication with modern coronary stent platforms–time to think beyond deliverability? EuroIntervention 2011;7(7):872–7.

29. Abdel-Wahab M, Sulimov DS, Kassner G, et al. Longitudinal deformation of contemporary coronary stents: an integrated analysis of clinical experience and observations from the bench. J Interv Cardiol 2012;25(6):576–85.

30. Ormiston JA, Webber B, Ubod B, et al. Stent longitudinal strength assessed using point compression: insights from a second-generation, clinically related bench test. Circ Cardiovasc Interv 2014;7(1):62–9.

31. Ormiston JA, Webber B, Webster MW. Stent longitudinal integrity bench insights into a clinical problem. JACC Cardiovasc Interv 2011;4(12):1310–7.

32. Bartorelli AL, Andreini D, Pontone G, et al. Stent longitudinal distortion: strut separation (pseudofracture) and strut compression ("concertina" effect). EuroIntervention 2012;8(2):290–1.

33. Shannon J, Latib A, Takagi K, et al. Procedural trauma risks longitudinal shortening of the promus element stent platform. Catheter Cardiovasc Interv 2013;81(5):810–7.

34. Pitney M, Pitney K, Jepson N, et al. Major stent deformation/pseudofracture of 7 Crown Endeavor/Micro Driver stent platform: incidence and causative factors. EuroIntervention 2011;7(2):256–62.

35. Inaba S, Weisz G, Kobayashi N, et al. Prevalence and anatomical features of acute longitudinal stent deformation: an intravascular ultrasound study. Catheter Cardiovasc Interv 2014;84(3):388–96.

36. Rigattieri S, Sciahbasi A, Loschiavo P. The clinical spectrum of longitudinal deformation of coronary stents: from a mere angiographic finding to a severe complication. J Invasive Cardiol 2013;25(5): E101–5.

37. Carrozza JP Jr, Hosley SE, Cohen DJ, et al. In vivo assessment of stent expansion and recoil in normal porcine coronary arteries: differential outcome by stent design. Circulation 1999;100(7):756–60.

38. Hong MK, Park SW, Lee CW, et al. Intravascular ultrasound comparison of chronic recoil among different stent designs. Am J Cardiol 1999;84(10): 1247–50. A8.

39. Costa MA, Sabate M, Kay IP, et al. Three-dimensional intravascular ultrasonic volumetric quantification of stent recoil and neointimal formation of two new generation tubular stents. Am J Cardiol 2000; 85(2):135–9.

40. Garcia LA, Hosley SE, Baim DS, et al. In vivo assessment of stent recoil in normal porcine arteries: evaluation of contemporary stent designs. Catheter Cardiovasc Interv 2001;53(2):277–80.

41. Tanimoto S, Bruining N, van Domburg RT, et al. Late stent recoil of the bioabsorbable everolimus-eluting coronary stent and its relationship with plaque morphology. J Am Coll Cardiol 2008;52(20): 1616–20.

42. He Y, Maehara A, Mintz GS, et al. Intravascular ultrasound assessment of cobalt chromium versus stainless steel drug-eluting stent expansion. Am J Cardiol 2010;105(9):1272–5.

43. Koo BK, Waseda K, Ako J, et al. Incidence of diffuse and focal chronic stent recoil after implantation of current generation bare-metal and drug-eluting stents. Int J Cardiol 2010;144(1):132–4.

44. Ormiston JA, Serruys PW, Regar E, et al. A bioabsorbable everolimus-eluting coronary stent system for patients with single de-novo coronary artery lesions (ABSORB): a prospective open-label trial. Lancet 2008;371(9616):899–907.

45. Nakatani S, Onuma Y, Ishibashi Y, et al. Incidence and potential mechanism of resolved, persistent and newly acquired malapposition three days after implantation of self-expanding or balloon-expandable stents in a STEMI population: insights from optical coherence tomography in the APPOSITION II study. EuroIntervention 2015;11(7):885–94.

46. Ota T, Ishii H, Sumi T, et al. Impact of coronary stent designs on acute stent recoil. J Cardiol 2014;64(5):347–52.

47. Williams PD, Appleby CE, Chowdhary S, et al. Double stenting: a method for treating acute stent recoil and luminal filling defects. EuroIntervention 2011;6(7):846–53.

48. Hong MK, Park SW, Lee CW, et al. Long-term outcomes of minor plaque prolapsed within stents documented with intravascular ultrasound. Catheter Cardiovasc Interv 2000;51(1):22–6.

49. Kim SW, Mintz GS, Ohlmann P, et al. Frequency and severity of plaque prolapse within cypher and

taxus stents as determined by sequential intravascular ultrasound analysis. Am J Cardiol 2006;98(9): 1206–11.

50. Futamatsu H, Sabaté M, Angiolillo DJ, et al. Characterization of plaque prolapse after drug-eluting stent implantation in diabetic patients: a three-dimensional volumetric intravascular ultrasound outcome study. J Am Coll Cardiol 2006;48(6): 1139–45.

51. Gonzalo N, Serruys PW, Okamura T, et al. Optical coherence tomography assessment of the acute effects of stent implantation on the vessel wall: a systematic quantitative approach. Heart 2009;95(23): 1913–9.

52. Hong YJ, Jeong MH, Choi YH, et al. Impact of tissue prolapse after stent implantation on short- and long-term clinical outcomes in patients with acute myocardial infarction: an intravascular ultrasound analysis. Int J Cardiol 2013;166(3):646–51.

53. Hong YJ, Jeong MH, Ahn Y, et al. Plaque prolapse after stent implantation in patients with acute myocardial infarction: an intravascular ultrasound analysis. JACC Cardiovasc Imaging 2008;1(4):489–97.

54. Sohn J, Hur SH, Kim IC, et al. A comparison of tissue prolapse with optical coherence tomography and intravascular ultrasound after drug-eluting stent implantation. Int J Cardiovasc Imaging 2015; 31(1):21–9.

55. Stone GW, Abizaid A, Silber S, et al. Prospective, randomized, multicenter evaluation of a polyethylene terephthalate micronet mesh-covered stent (MGuard) in ST-segment elevation myocardial infarction: the MASTER trial. J Am Coll Cardiol 2012;60(19):1975–84.

56. Fernandez-Cisnal A, Cid-Álvarez B, Álvarez-Álvarez B, et al. Real world comparison of the MGuard stent versus the bare metal stent for ST elevation myocardial infarction (the REWARD-MI study). Catheter Cardiovasc Interv 2015;85(1):E1–9.

57. Shen ZJ, Brugaletta S, Garcia-Garcia HM, et al. Comparison of plaque prolapse in consecutive patients treated with Xience V and Taxus Liberte stents. Int J Cardiovasc Imaging 2012;28(1):23–31.

58. Choi SY, Witzenbichler B, Maehara A, et al. Intravascular ultrasound findings of early stent thrombosis after primary percutaneous intervention in acute myocardial infarction: a harmonizing outcomes with revascularization and stents in acute myocardial infarction (HORIZONS-AMI) substudy. Circ Cardiovasc Interv 2011;4(3):239–47.

Moving?

Make sure your subscription moves with you!

To notify us of your new address, find your **Clinics Account Number** (located on your mailing label above your name), and contact customer service at:

Email: journalscustomerservice-usa@elsevier.com

800-654-2452 (subscribers in the U.S. & Canada)
314-447-8871 (subscribers outside of the U.S. & Canada)

Fax number: 314-447-8029

Elsevier Health Sciences Division
Subscription Customer Service
3251 Riverport Lane
Maryland Heights, MO 63043

*To ensure uninterrupted delivery of your subscription, please notify us at least 4 weeks in advance of move.

ELSEVIER

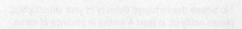

Printed and bound by CPI Group (UK) Ltd, Croydon, CR0 4YY

03/10/2024

01040302-0009